Evaluating HIV/AIDS Health Promotion

Evaluating HIV/AIDS Health Promotion

A Resource for HIV/AIDS Health Promotion Workers
in Statutory and Voluntary Organisations

by PETER AGGLETON
DIANE MOODY
ANDREA YOUNG

with exercises by GRAZ KOWSZUN

and illustrations by TAMSIN WILTON

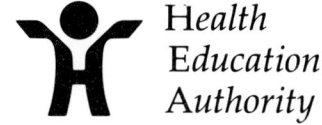

Published in 1992

Health Education Authority
Hamilton House
Mabledon Place
London WC1H 9TX

ISBN 1 85448 258 0

© Health Education Authority 1992

Typeset by DP Photosetting, Aylesbury, Bucks
Printed by Scotprint Ltd

Contents

	Introduction	1
	Assessing your current knowledge and attitudes	2
	Making a start	3
1.	**What is evaluation?**	**7**
	Introduction	7
	The context of monitoring and evaluation	7
	Monitoring and evaluation – some terms defined	10
	Managing the evaluation process	14
	The uses of evaluation	15
	Conclusions	16
2.	**Planning evaluation**	**17**
	Introduction	17
	Setting aims and objectives	17
	Why evaluate?	20
	What should be evaluated?	23
	Who evaluates?	25
	When to evaluate?	28
	The scope of evaluation	29
	Conclusions	30
3.	**How to evaluate – process evaluation**	**32**
	Introduction	32
	Eliciting participants' views	32
	Record keeping	42
	Conclusions	44
4.	**How to evaluate – outcome evaluation**	**45**
	Introduction	45
	Indicators	45
	Research designs in evaluation	47
	Value for money	55
	Conclusions	58

5. Producing evaluation reports — 59

Introduction — 59
Analysing information — 59
Interpreting results — 62
Writing reports — 62
Conclusions — 67

6. Using evaluation — 68

Introduction — 68
Influencing policy — 69
Influencing personal and professional life — 70
Conclusions — 71

Appendix — 73
Constructing a questionnaire — 73
Wording questions — 74
Analysing the results — 75

References — 77

Acknowledgements

Evaluating HIV/AIDS Health Promotion has been developed by Peter Aggleton, Project Director (Goldsmiths' College, University of London), Graz Kowszun (Goldsmiths' College, University of London), Diane Moody (Bristol Polytechnic) and Andrea Young (Health Education Authority). They have been supported by an Advisory Group consisting of Jo Adams (Sheffield AIDS Education Project), Ann Boardman (Southend Health Authority), Kate Butcher (Leeds Western Health Authority), Alan Glanz (Health Education Authority) and Greg Lucas (NW Thames HIV Project, London). Secretarial assistance was provided by Heather Jones (Bristol Polytechnic) and Helen Thomas (Goldsmiths' College, University of London).

The following have also provided advice, encouragement and support: Elaine Chase (Learning about AIDS Project, Goldsmiths' College, University of London), Hilary Dixon, Michele Lazarus (NW Thames HIV Project, London), Frankie Lynch (Terrence Higgins Trust), Sonya Welch (Goldsmiths' College, University of London), Mark Whittaker (Goldsmiths' College, University of London) and Tamsin Wilton (Bristol Polytechnic).

Introduction

- **Assessing your current knowledge and attitudes**
- **Making a start**

As part of the support offered to health authorities, local authorities and voluntary sector organisations, the Health Education Authority (HEA) has developed a range of resources to assist local HIV/AIDS workers in monitoring and evaluating their work. These include an HIV/AIDS and Sexual Health Programme paper, *Monitoring and Evaluating Local HIV/AIDS Programmes* by Diane Moody, Andrea Young, Peter Aggleton, Mukesh Kapila and Maryan Pye (HEA, 1991) and a book *Does it Work? Perspectives on the Evaluation of HIV/AIDS Health Promotion* edited by Peter Aggleton, Andrea Young, Diane Moody, Mukesh Kapila and Maryan Pye (HEA, 1992) which contains case studies of monitoring and evaluating HIV/AIDS health promotion.

Evaluating HIV/AIDS Health Promotion is an additional resource for those undertaking local evaluation. It introduces key concepts and terminology, and provides guidance on how to set up and run an evaluation programme. The material has been organised so that it is accessible to a broad spectrum of people involved in HIV/AIDS health promotion, and a range of exercises are provided to help you to acquire the necessary skills. These exercises can be carried out either individually or as part of a professional development exercise involving colleagues.

To promote the use of the manual, there will be a dissemination programme throughout 1992. For further details of this programme, which will be organised on a regional basis, contact Mark Whittaker or Peter Aggleton, Health and Education Research Unit, Faculty of Education, Goldsmiths' College, University of London, Lewisham Way, London SE14 6NW; Tel: 081-694 2033, Fax: 081-694 0485.

Assessing your current knowledge and attitudes

Before looking at the processes involved in monitoring and evaluation, it may be helpful to identify your current knowledge of, and attitudes towards, evaluation.

Exercise 1 **Self-assessment**

Aim To help you to identify your attitude towards evaluation and your confidence in carrying it out.

A. How would you rate yourself as an evaluator of HIV/AIDS health promotion on a scale from 0 (very poor) through 5 (adequate) to 10 (excellent) in the following areas? Date and keep a copy of your response so that you can refer back to it later.

(i) Overall knowledge of evaluation. ☐

(ii) Knowing how to carry out evaluation and knowing which approaches to use in specific situations. ☐

(iii) Confidence that you have the necessary understanding to meet the evaluation needs of your present post. ☐

B. How would you rate your current attitude to evaluation on a scale of 0 (very low opinion) through 5 (sometimes useful) to 10 (essential)? ☐

Exercise 2 **Current knowledge and attitudes towards evaluation**

Aim To help you to assess your current knowledge of evaluation and your attitudes towards it.

Take ten minutes to produce patterned notes on the topic of evaluation. First, write down the word 'EVALUATION' in the centre of a page. Then draw lines branching out from it to represent your thoughts and ideas. Do not worry about order, emphasis and organisation – allow the pattern to unfold organically. It is a good idea to use capital letters, to print words on lines and to ensure that each line within a branch is connected to another. Shown opposite are the patterned notes one person generated when asked to write down her initial thoughts about

Introduction

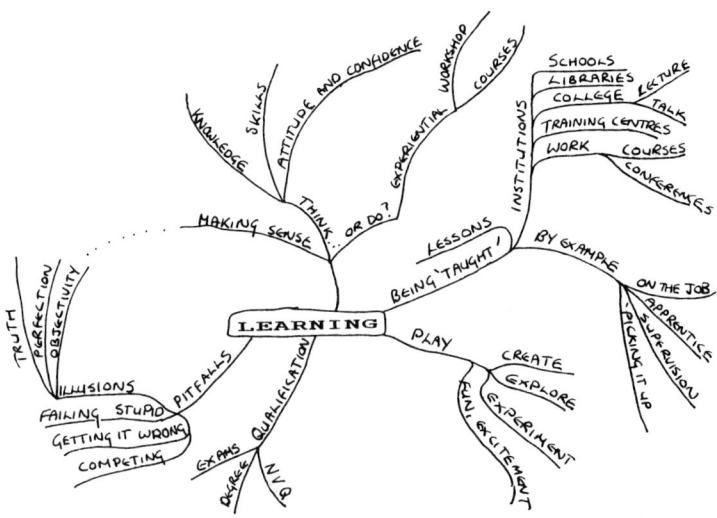

the topic 'LEARNING'. (For more information about making patterned notes, you might like to read Tony Buzan's book *Use Your Head*, BBC Publications, 1974.)

Once you have completed the exercise, look at your patterned notes. What is your overall impression? Are your notes entirely factual or have you also made reference to your attitudes and feelings? Are there any responses or patterns that surprise you? Does the density or complexity of the pattern vary from side to side? If so, does this suggest anything about areas of particular interest to you, or does it point to gaps in your confidence and skills? Date and keep your notes safely, as you will need to refer to them later.

Making a start

It may not be necessary for you to read and to study this book from cover to cover. The chart on pages 4–6 has been designed to help you to use this resource practically. In the process of identifying what you already know about evaluation in Exercise 2, you may have recognised some gaps or further learning needs. Other areas may come to light as you take on more evaluation tasks at work. The chart is intended to direct you to the most relevant parts of the book, depending on your interests and needs.

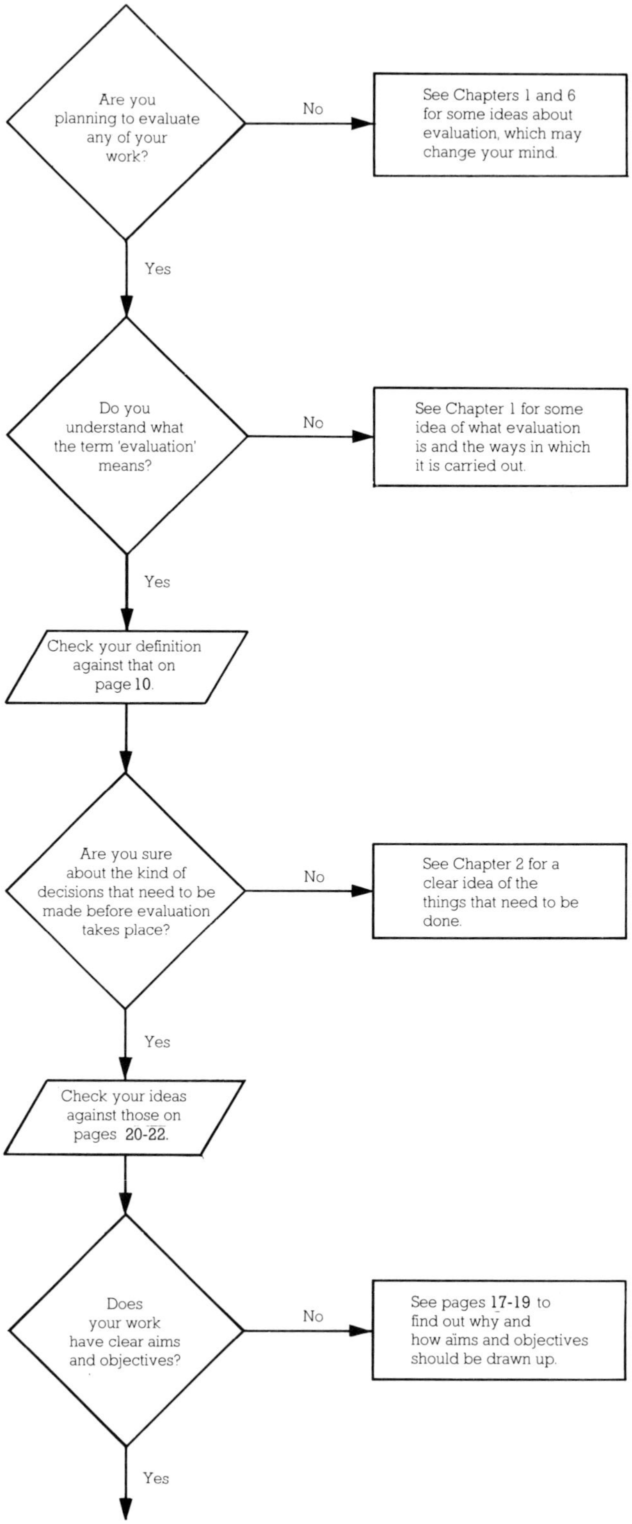

Evaluating HIV/AIDS health promotion

```
         ┌─────────────────┐
         │ Are you         │    No    ┌──────────────────────┐
         │ planning to     │─────────▶│ See Chapters 1 and 6 │
         │ evaluate any of │          │ for some ideas about │
         │ your work?      │          │ evaluation, which may│
         └─────────────────┘          │ change your mind.    │
                 │                    └──────────────────────┘
                 │ Yes
                 ▼
         ┌─────────────────┐
         │ Do you          │    No    ┌──────────────────────┐
         │ understand what │─────────▶│ See Chapter 1 for some│
         │ the term        │          │ idea of what evaluation│
         │ 'evaluation'    │          │ is and the ways in which│
         │ means?          │          │ it is carried out.   │
         └─────────────────┘          └──────────────────────┘
                 │ Yes
                 ▼
         ┌─────────────────┐
         │ Check your      │
         │ definition      │
         │ against that on │
         │ page 10.        │
         └─────────────────┘
                 │
                 ▼
         ┌─────────────────┐
         │ Are you sure    │    No    ┌──────────────────────┐
         │ about the kind  │─────────▶│ See Chapter 2 for a  │
         │ of decisions    │          │ clear idea of the    │
         │ that need to be │          │ things that need to be│
         │ made before     │          │ done.                │
         │ evaluation      │          └──────────────────────┘
         │ takes place?    │
         └─────────────────┘
                 │ Yes
                 ▼
         ┌─────────────────┐
         │ Check your ideas│
         │ against those on│
         │ pages 20-22.    │
         └─────────────────┘
                 │
                 ▼
         ┌─────────────────┐
         │ Does your work  │    No    ┌──────────────────────┐
         │ have clear aims │─────────▶│ See pages 17-19 to   │
         │ and objectives? │          │ find out why and     │
         │                 │          │ how aims and objectives│
         │                 │          │ should be drawn up.  │
         └─────────────────┘          └──────────────────────┘
                 │ Yes
                 ▼
```

Introduction

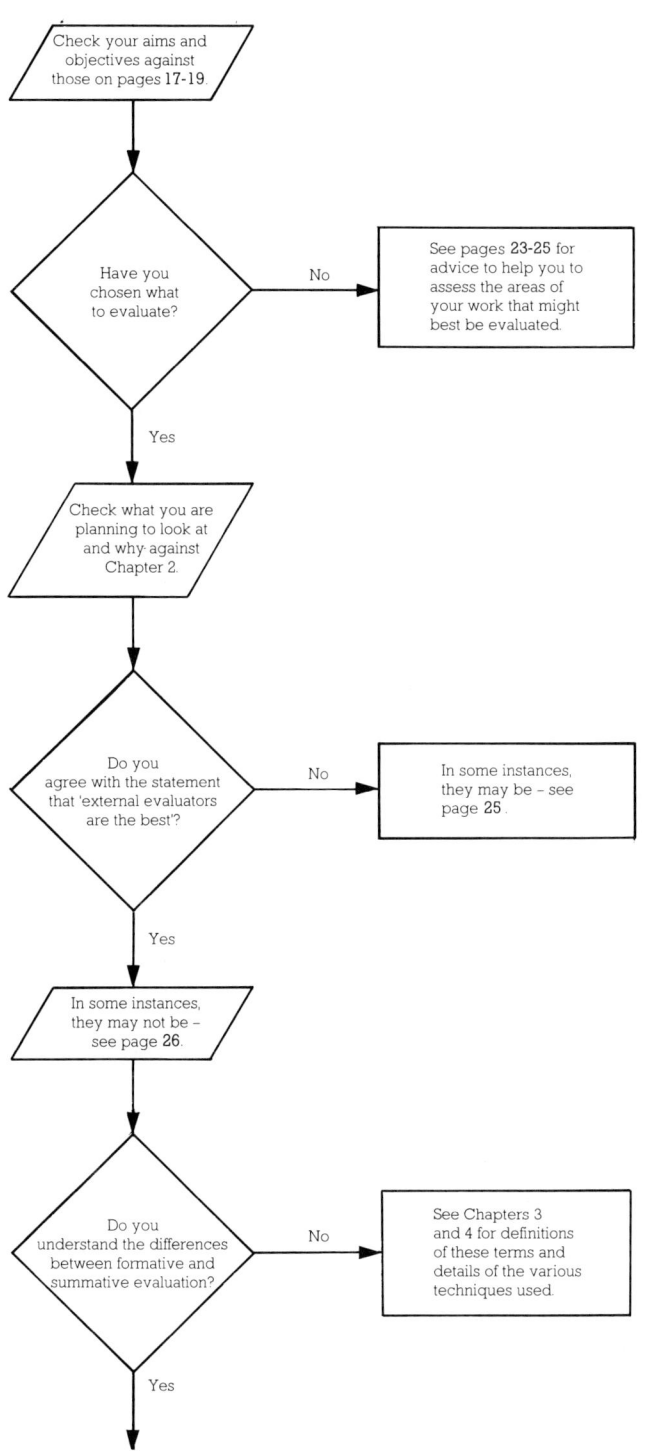

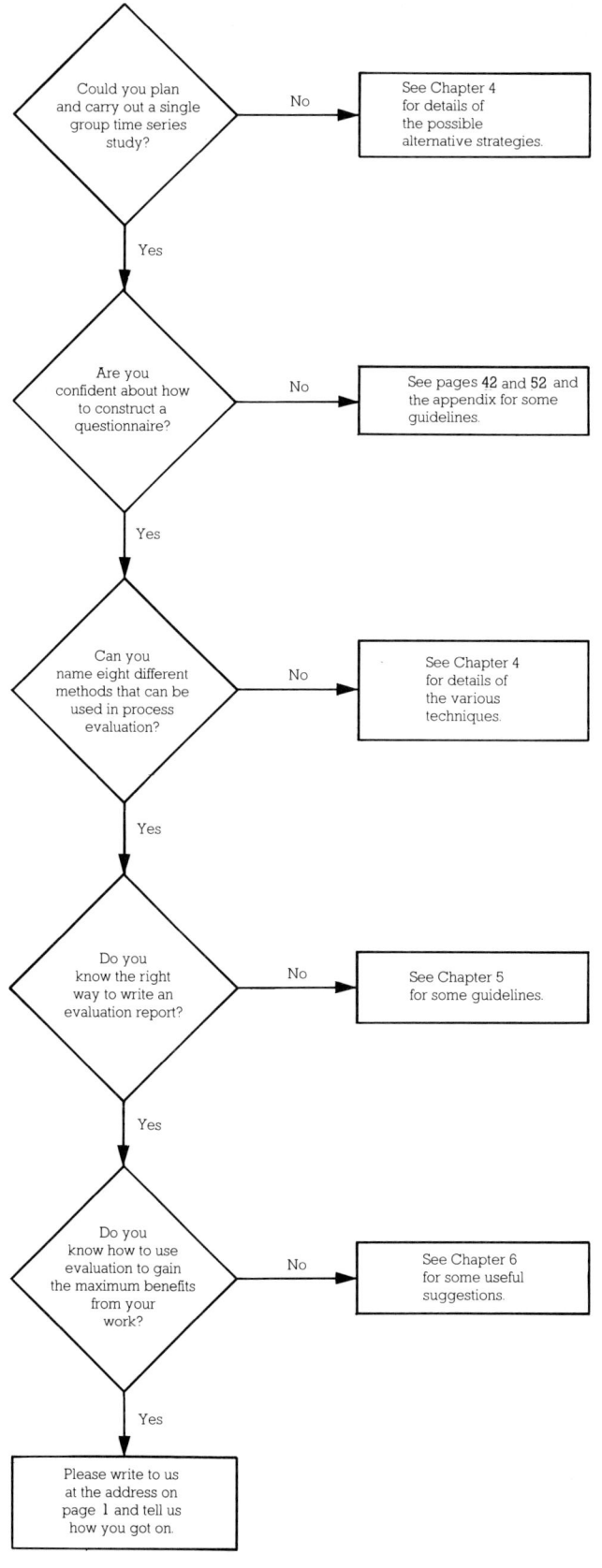

CHAPTER 1

What is evaluation?

- Context • Monitoring and evaluation defined
- Managing the evaluation process • Uses of evaluation

Introduction

Health educators and health promoters are being increasingly called upon to monitor and to evaluate their work. Sometimes the pressure for this comes from those who sponsor or fund particular projects; sometimes it comes from employing authorities who want to find out whether resources are being used effectively; and sometimes it comes from health educators and health promoters themselves who want to know whether a particular initiative has been successful, and if so, why.

These pressures are particularly acute in the field of HIV/AIDS health promotion, where health authorities and local authorities are keen to find out whether or not funds have been well spent, and where voluntary groups and HIV/AIDS service organisations are keen to identify the health promotion strategies that work to best advantage. It is in response to these demands that this manual has been produced as part of the Health Education Authority's work to support the monitoring and evaluation of local HIV/AIDS programmes. The aim is to demystify seemingly obscure and technical procedures – the preserve of scientists and 'experts' of one kind and another – and to offer health educators and health promoters guidance in adopting the most appropriate techniques.

In this introductory chapter, we will:

- discuss the context in which monitoring and evaluation take place;
- define some key terms;
- describe some of the uses of monitoring and evaluation in HIV/AIDS work.

The context of monitoring and evaluation

Monitoring and evaluation rarely, if ever, take place in a vacuum. They occur because people believe that it is important to monitor and to evaluate health promotion work, and to satisfy certain goals. On the positive side, these goals can include the desire to show that health promotion is being successful, the need to demonstrate to others that resources are being well allocated, and the hope of identifying the most effective ways of reaching certain groups. On the more negative side, monitoring and evaluation may be carried out to provide the evidence needed to close down a project, to demonstrate that a project's aims and intentions are not being adhered to, or to justify the reallocation of resources to other fields of work. Ideally, however, monitoring and evaluation are carried out to find out what is going on and to ascertain why certain outcomes have been achieved.

The interests of funders, policy makers and sponsors, the interests of health educators and health promoters themselves, and the interests of client groups all impinge upon monitoring and evaluation. They establish the *political* context within which monitoring and evaluation take place, and they influence the ways in which findings are subsequently interpreted. Broader political issues also surround the monitoring and evaluation of HIV/AIDS health promotion, and these arise from the fact that topics such as injecting drug use, sex, sexuality and safer sex arouse strong feelings – feelings that are often linked to religious and moral standpoints. Values and beliefs are therefore likely to be reflected in the calls for monitoring and evaluation, and may influence the kind of data that is collected and the way the data are interpreted. For example, if it is believed that the aim of HIV/AIDS health promotion should be to stop people injecting drugs, rather than enabling them to inject safely, data on the number of people who have ceased to inject following an intervention would have to be collected. An alternative approach that focused on harm minimisation might be satisfied by the collection of data on the number of people coming into contact with and using the services provided by a syringe and needle exchange.

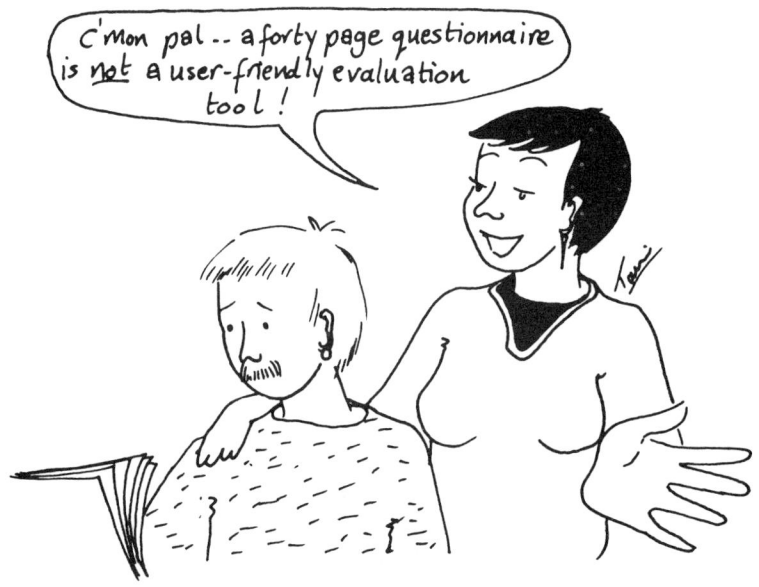

A rather different set of contextual factors needs to be taken into account when monitoring and evaluating HIV/AIDS work. Contemporary mass media reports about HIV/AIDS, statements by politicians and religious leaders, and fears triggered by scientific uncertainty about the nature of HIV establish and reinforce popular beliefs – beliefs that can disorientate the effects of HIV/AIDS health promotion activities, and thus bias the findings from an evaluation of these activities. For example, evaluation data collected following a week-long local HIV/AIDS health promotion programme pointing out what can be done to prevent the heterosexual transmission of HIV may be skewed if there have been concurrent reports in the tabloid press that suggest that heterosexual transmission is impossible. Similarly, one-off television documentaries that present as 'fact' minority opinions about HIV/AIDS can seriously affect the impact of HIV/AIDS health promotion activity. When evaluating local work, these possible influences need to be taken into account.

Exercise 3 **Evaluation – shadow and light**

Aim To help you to identify the positive and negative aspects of evaluation.

- What are your hopes and positive expectations about evaluation?
- On the other hand, what are your fears and negative expectations?

If you see yourself as a logical 'left-side-of-the-brain' thinker, you might like to write down answers to these questions in a list. You may also find completing the following sentences helpful in generating your list: 'At best, evaluation can be . . .' and 'At worst, evaluation can be . . .'

If you prefer a more lateral and creative 'right-side-of-the-brain' approach, try letting your imagination offer a response by describing, or drawing, this thing/activity called evaluation. Having come up with some images, take some time to reflect on them. Why might you have chosen particular forms or characteristics? What do the shapes, sizes, textures and colours suggest about your attitudes to evaluation? What feelings do they convey?

It is important to acknowledge positive *and* negative expectations, and hopes and fears about evaluation at the outset.

Some of these may be more realistic than others, and some may be more or less central to the process of evaluation itself. There is no doubt that evaluation has both an 'upside' and a 'downside'. By considering what can be controlled, avoided or built into the process of evaluation, we empower ourselves. By acknowledging the reality of the situation in which we work, we can identify the limits of our control and act accordingly, maximising positive outcomes and minimising negative ones.

Monitoring and evaluation – some terms defined

Monitoring has been defined by the World Health Organisation as 'the process of follow-up of activities to ensure that they are proceeding according to plan.'(1) It involves an ongoing collection of data concerning the progress of a health promotion activity. These data may then be used to fine-tune that activity.

Evaluation, on the other hand, is the 'determination of the effectiveness, efficiency and acceptability of a planned intervention in achieving stated objectives.'(2) In HIV/AIDS work, as in other kinds of health promotion, two types of evaluation are often distinguished – outcome evaluation and process evaluation.

Exercise 4 **Assessing progress or effectiveness?**

Aim To help you to distinguish more clearly between monitoring (progress) and evaluation (effectiveness).

Study the following statements and mark each with a 'P' if you consider it contains information relevant to assessing the *progress* of an activity. If, on the other hand, you consider it relevant to assessing the *effectiveness* of the activity, mark it with an 'E'. If you are not sure about the information, do not mark the statement at all – sometimes it is difficult to decide between progress and effectivenesss if it is not clear what activity is under consideration and what its objectives are.

A. Twenty-seven awareness days have now been run and a total of 317 local residents and workers have attended. ☐

B. Post-training questionnaires reveal that most respondents feel more confident and knowledgeable about how to negotiate safer sex. ☐

C. Following a month-long advertising campaign, a survey of randomly selected voluntary sector projects in the district has revealed that two-thirds of respondents knew that 1990 World AIDS Day focused on women and that free information packs were available from the library. ☐

D. 'As a supervisor of HIV counsellors, I am aware that some gay men and also women are having unprotected sex with their HIV antibody-positive partners out of desperation over how to show their love. Those counsellors who encourage the client to explore the complex feelings without judgement and panic are much more effective in getting people to change their behaviour. I've noticed that those counsellors who reprimand the folly of the client tend not to see the client again.' ☐

E. Statistics have revealed that 17% of residents sampled in Healthtown know of the existence of the local AIDS helpline and either have the number or are confident they could get it if necessary. However, only 0.3% of these residents admitted to having used it. ☐

Outcome or summative evaluation, as the name suggests, is concerned with the outputs and outcomes of health promotion activities. It identifies the effectiveness of an activity in meeting its predefined objectives. For example, if a local leaflet campaign aims to increase public knowledge about the ways in which HIV is and is not transmitted, an outcome evaluation of this initiative would aim to examine changes in knowledge levels before and after the intervention.

Process or formative evaluation, on the other hand, offers feedback on what took place when a particular activity or programme was implemented. It may, for example, provide information on the roles of participants or stakeholders (i.e. those who have an interest in the success of the activity), the organisational model that underpinned the activity, the history of the activity, and the social and political context in which it took place. Instead of providing feedback on the results of an activity, it tries to explain *how* these outcomes were brought about. Process evaluation of a training workshop for HIV/AIDS counsellors, for example, might focus on patterns of communication and group dynamics throughout the course.

Exercise 5 **Evaluation – collecting useful information**

Aim To identify the kind of information that will be useful in carrying out an evaluation.

Which of the following items are useful data for evaluation purposes? Tick those that you consider may be useful and make some notes about what the data might demonstrate about the HIV/AIDS health promotion activity in question. (Note that it is only possible to guess at the relevance of data without knowing what activity and what objectives are being evaluated.) What else might you need to consider to assess whether the data are relevant for evaluation purposes (e.g. limitations of the information, importance of time-scale)?

Data	Comments	Useful?
Client contact sheets from an HIV counselling service, showing pseudonym, age, sex, ethnic group and sexual orientation of attenders.		
Trainers talking in a car on the way back to the office about how the latest of their quarterly sessions at a youth club had gone. 'Those three lads in the navy/white jackets were so disruptive with their heckling.' 'Yes, and did you notice all that anti-gay graffiti that's recently appeared?'		
A daily 'headcount', a stock count of condoms and 'safer injecting' leaflets, and a month's worth of food shopping bills from a day centre for people with a recent history of injecting drug use.		
Needle exchange worker explaining to an interviewer that while clients said they never shared syringes and therefore did not need bleach, when supplies of small bottles of bleach were left in the toilets, they had to be restocked every 2–3 days.		
Graph showing how many of a random sample of local 16–20 years olds recently surveyed claimed to have started a new romantic relationship in the last six months and the proportion who claimed not to have had penetrative sex in this time. This graph is set alongside similar graphs for 1988 and 1990.		
Outreach worker's diary entry: 'Di talked to me again and was defensively curious about drug rehabilitation hostels. "Haven't injected for months now and maybe it's time to leave gear right out?" she said. Arranged to go to street agency together tomorrow but did not appear.'		
Telephone log sheet for first day of each of the last 16 months from a local AIDS helpline.		
Stock reports from condom company showing that orders in town X for 1990 were down by 14% in comparison with 1987 figures but still 43% up on the average figures for 1975–84.		

What is evaluation? 13

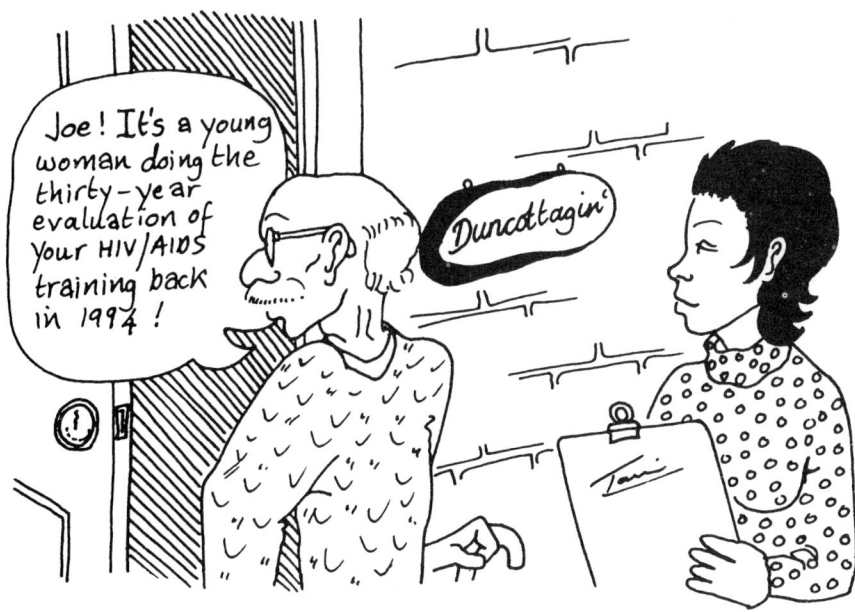

When carrying out an evaluation of an HIV/AIDS health promotion activity, it is often useful to draw a distinction between short- and long-term evaluation. Many of the goals in this kind of work cannot be achieved in the short term. A period of time may be necessary before they can be realised. It is clearly less than reasonable to expect people to switch to safer sex after watching a five-minute video on the subject. While the video and the issues it addresses may trigger the process of behaviour change, other interventions may be necessary to provide individuals with support as they begin to modify their behaviour. While *short-term* (or interim) evaluation may pick up the initial motivation towards behaviour change, *long-term* evaluation will be necessary to assess whether or not it takes place.

It is also important to consider *unintended consequences* when evaluating HIV/AIDS health promotion. Thus, in Britain today, an intervention that focuses uncritically on the 'origins' of HIV may unintentionally reinforce racism, and an intervention that looks at the groups most affected by HIV/AIDS may unintentionally reinforce anti-gay attitudes and prejudice towards injecting drug users. Knowing in advance how best to assess these unintended consequences can be difficult, but evaluators should keep an open mind when going about their work, remaining alert to the possibility that health promotion interventions may generate a variety of outcomes, not all of them intended.

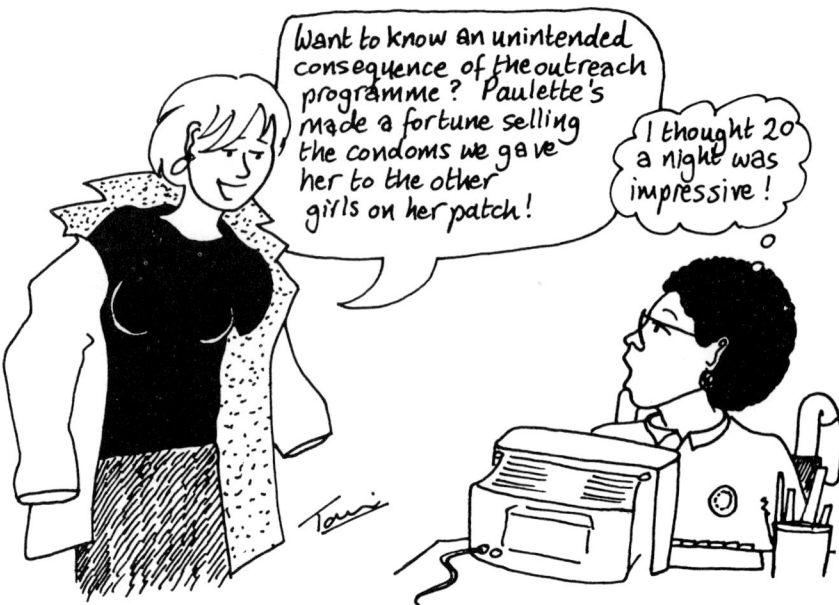

Managing the evaluation process

When planning the evaluation of an HIV/AIDS health promotion activity, it is important to consider how the process is to be managed. In particular, decisions will need to be made about:

- The type of contract that exists between the evaluator(s), the funders/sponsors of the evaluation and those whose work is being evaluated. Is it verbal or written? How was this negotiated? What scope is there for revision?
- Who will collect data, when and from whom?
- The type of data that will be collected. Will this be in number form (quantitative) or will it be more descriptive (qualitative)?
- The kind of confidentiality that respondents can expect. Will their responses be reported directly, or will they be paraphrased or presented as part of a broader summary?
- Who will manage the evaluation and keep regular checks on progress, finance, etc.?
- The 'ownership' of the data. Will this rest with respondents, the research team, the funders, the project's steering group or jointly between all of these parties?

Once evaluation is underway, there will be a need for regular feedback from the evaluation team to those whose work is being evaluated. There are advantages in adopting a *transactional* approach to evaluation, whereby initial findings are presented for comment, modification and amendment as necessary. In this way, findings from the evaluation can be made more reliable (in the sense that more people may agree with them) and possibly more valid (in the sense that they may more accurately reflect what was going on). Transactional approaches do, however, have disadvantages, in that it may be difficult to reconcile different 'interpretations' of what happened. They may also be unduly influenced by the views of powerful and influential individuals.(3)

A special advisory or steering group may be set up to receive findings from the evaluation and to comment upon them. If this is the case, it is important to define in advance what the responsibilities of this group will be, how it will operate and to whom it will be accountable (funders/sponsors, those whose work was being evaluated, broader community interests, etc.).

The uses of evaluation

Findings from an evaluation of HIV/AIDS health promotion work can be used in a variety of ways. They can be used to assess what has been achieved, to measure the impact of a health promotion initiative, to identify its strengths and weaknesses in meeting particular goals, to aid future planning, to judge cost effectiveness and to justify decision making. These, and further uses, are discussed in more depth in the following Chapter 2.

More generally, evaluation can also be used to influence self and group development, to suggest alternative ways in which HIV/AIDS health promotion should take place, and to influence the development and implementation of policy. These and other similar uses are examined in Chapter 6.

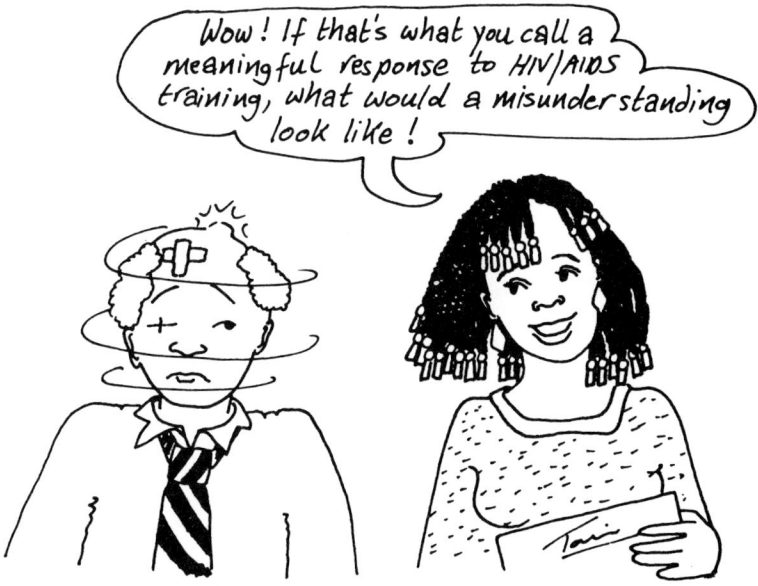

Conclusions

Monitoring and evaluation can sometimes seem difficult and highly technical processes, involving procedures that can only be carried out by 'experts' of one kind or another. This preliminary chapter has tried to show that this is not the case, but that there is a 'language' to evaluation that involves the use of technical terms. The procedures involved are in principle not all that difficult. In the remainder of this book, we look in depth at some of these techniques and offer guidance on how they can be implemented when it comes to monitoring and evaluating local HIV/AIDS work.

CHAPTER 2 Planning evaluation

- Setting aims and objectives • Why evaluate?
- What should be evaluated? • Who evaluates?
- When to evaluate? • The scope of evaluation

Introduction

Evaluation can sometimes seem a complex and difficult process. Often, the greatest difficulty is knowing where to start. It is important, first, to specify the aims and objectives of an HIV/AIDS health promotion activity. Planning what needs to be done is the second important step. This need not necessarily be a difficult task, but planning requires giving careful consideration to questions such as 'Why evaluate?', 'What should be evaluated?', 'Who should do the evaluation?' and 'When should evaluation take place?'. It is also important to set limits to the scope of the evaluation.

Setting aims and objectives

Setting clear and precise aims and objectives for an HIV/AIDS health promotion activity is the important first step in evaluation, although there is often some degree of confusion over what these terms mean. An *aim* normally describes the general intent or outcome of an activity. For example, the aim of a needle exchange scheme may be 'to reduce HIV infection among injecting drug users in Greater Knaseby and the surrounding area'. Usually, and because of its general nature, only one aim is stated. An *objective*, on the other hand, is much more specific, and any one aim may give rise to a number of specific objectives. For example, typical objectives of a needle exchange scheme could be: (a) 'to ensure the availability of needles and syringes to an identified client group'; (b) 'to provide information and advice on safer sex and safer injecting behaviour'; (c) 'to establish an easily recognised, accessible and user-friendly service'; (d) 'to provide a safe place for the disposal of used injecting equipment'; and (e) 'to promote easy access to counselling and treatment services for those concerned about their drug use and considering change'.

To offer another example, whereas the aim of an outreach project with men who have sex with men might be 'to encourage safer sex among men who cottage in Lower Braithwaite', the objectives of such a project may be: (a) 'to produce a leaflet providing safer sex information suitable to the needs of men who

18 *Evaluating HIV/AIDS health promotion*

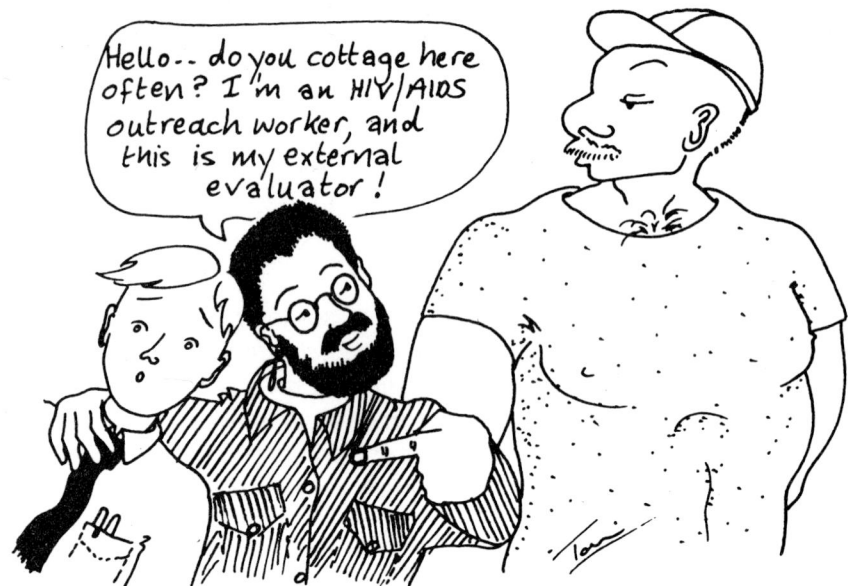

cottage'; (b) 'to make contact with as many individuals as possible who may be engaged in high risk behaviour'; (c) 'to provide advice and information on HIV/AIDS'; and (d) 'to act as an access point to the local genito-urinary medicine clinic'.

Aims and objectives have a particularly important part to play in evaluation. By setting well-defined aims and objectives that identify what an activity is expected to achieve, it is easier to know what to evaluate. Aims and objectives thereby point to what an evaluation may attempt to measure. Once a clear set of objectives has been defined, the success of an activity may be gauged by examining the extent to which these objectives have been met.

Exercise 6 **The aims and objectives of an activity**

Aim To help you to distinguish clearly between the aims and objectives of an HIV/AIDS health promotion activity.

A. Choose an HIV/AIDS health promotion project with which you are familiar and *either* obtain a list of its aims and objectives *or* write down what you think they may be.

B. Examine each of the objectives in your list closely and reword it if necessary using the mnemonic ST CRAVE:

Singular – have you allocated just one task/function to each objective?
 e.g. To explain the difference between HIV and AIDS.

Time-scale – has the time-scale been clearly identified?
> e.g. To run regular two-day AIDS awareness courses until July 1992, by which time 60% of local public sector workers should have attended.

Clear – is the objective expressed in concrete and specific terms, with no ambiguities?
> e.g. To offer a free and confidential needle exchange service that is open all year from 4 pm to 10 pm, Thursday to Monday.

Realistic – can the objective be achieved within available resources of time, energy, money, knowledge, etc.? Is it possible to manage/organise?
> e.g. However laudable it may be to wish to provide a counsellor of the same sex, sexuality and ethnic background as the client, how would you meet a request for, say, a South Pacific bisexual woman counsellor?

Appropriate – does the objective fit with the project's aim, politics, context, etc.?
> e.g. It would probably be inappropriate to run a daily drop-in service if you are a single worker with a broad range of responsibilities and no funding for relief cover.

Values – is it ethical and in line with the values of those involved and the stakeholders?
> e.g. Advertising a counselling service (as opposed to say 'a self-help and support service') when your personnel consists of three volunteers with HIV who have had no counselling training or experience is an example of unethical practice.

Evaluatable – will you be able to tell if you have done it and how?
> e.g. If one objective was to provide needle exchange facilities for 80% of local injecting drug users, how could you possibly know what progress you were making given the impossibility of knowing how many injecting drug users there are in your locality in the first place?

It is important, however, not to limit an evaluation to measuring only the extent to which objectives have been met. We also need to be aware that there may be unintended consequences of HIV/AIDS health promotion: things that were unexpected, but which may influence the overall success of an activity. For example, there may be increased police presence in the area of a needle exchange, or participants taking part in an HIV/AIDS course might subsequently provide information to their peers. In this case, it is important to know how such consequences come about as well as knowing what the outcomes are.

Why evaluate?

There are many reasons why it is important to evaluate HIV/AIDS health promotion activities. These include:

- To assess what an activity has achieved. This may be measured in terms of the extent to which its aims and objectives have been met.
- To measure the impact of the activity. Attempts may be made to measure the impact of the activity by, for example, assessing changes in knowledge or attitudes, or changes in behaviour.
- To monitor progress.
- To identify strengths and weaknesses. Evaluation should be able to identify failures as well as successes. It is important to learn from past experiences in order to strengthen future HIV/AIDS health promotion activities.
- To share experiences. A valuable aspect of evaluation is to reflect on past experience so that others can learn from this.
- To plan the way ahead. It may be important to collect information to be able to plan and manage activities in the future. This may include collecting information on participants' views and feelings so that an activity may be better tailored to the needs of those involved.

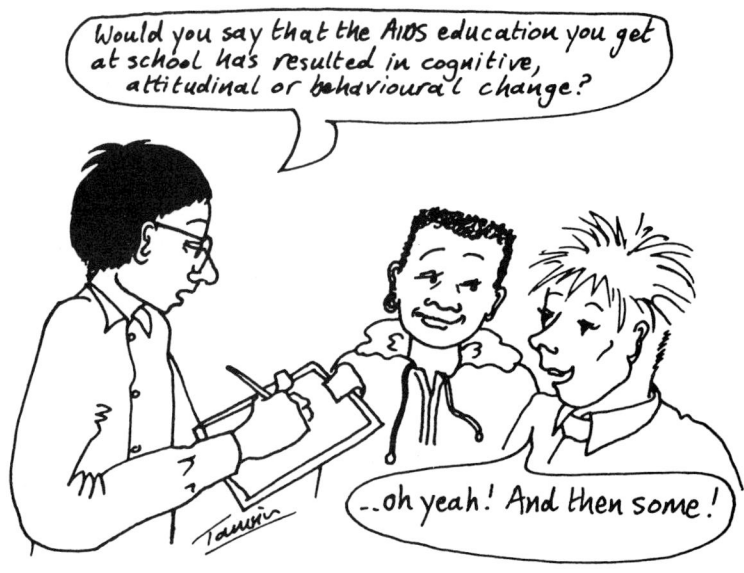

- To enhance staff development. It is important to use evaluation as part of team building. This can be done by valuing and validating the work of others, as well as yourself, thereby providing workers with a source of feedback and a chance to reflect.
- To judge cost effectiveness. It may be important to assess whether time, money and resources have been well spent.
- To justify decisions. It may be important to show the benefits of an activity in a situation where others may be uncertain or even hostile towards what is being undertaken. Managers and employers may be happier to provide time, resources and further funding for work if an evaluation clearly shows what has been achieved.

Exercise 7 **Why evaluate a project?**

Aim To help you to identify when it is appropriate to evaluate an HIV/AIDS health promotion project.

A. Choose a project with clearly stated aims and objectives and complete the following chart as fully as possible by considering the following:

- What short-term benefits (+) could arise from evaluation?
- What short-term costs (−) could arise from evaluation?
- What long-term benefits (+) could arise from evaluation?
- What long-term costs (−) could arise from evaluation?

Remember that evaluation can cover both what is achieved (outcomes) and how it is achieved (process).

B. Which of your lists is longer? In purely quantitative terms, do the costs outweigh the benefits or vice versa?

C. Some factors on your list may be more important than others. In terms of their significance (i.e. in qualitative terms), what is the balance between the costs and the benefits? Is it worth proceeding with an evaluation on this occasion?

D. Assuming it makes sense to evaluate, and you decide that an evaluation is worth doing, can you reduce any of the costs without jeopardising the evaluation as a whole? Or is it possible to introduce additional benefits to make the evaluation even more worthwhile?

Benefits and costs linked to the evaluation of an HIV/AIDS health promotion project

Name of project:			
Short-term		Long-term	
+	−	+	−

What should be evaluated?

Successful evaluation can provide a clear indication of the success and achievements of an HIV/AIDS health promotion activity, as well as useful information for decision making. Often, however, too much is expected of evaluation. The hope is that it will answer every possible question. But due to the constraints of time and resources, the scope of any one evaluation is limited, with the result that not all questions can be answered. The questions an evaluation asks, and the answers that it can be expected to provide, must therefore be carefully thought out and agreed in advance. It is important to recognise that evaluation may seek to do several things. First, it may look at the outputs and outcomes of the health promotion activity. Second, it may examine its nature or process. Third, and ideally, it may do all of these things.

It is often important to evaluate the *outputs* of an activity – that is, the products produced and the services provided. This kind of evaluation is a quantitative exercise and involves, for example, assessing how many people have been involved in a training activity, how many leaflets have been produced and how many calls have been made to an AIDS helpline in a fixed period of time.

An evaluation of an activity's achievements may also include questions about its *impact* or *outcomes*. Such an attempt to assess the effects of an activity is usually called *outcome evaluation* (see page 45). It may, for example, enquire whether the knowledge of those taking part in a training course has changed, whether those reading a leaflet have understood the

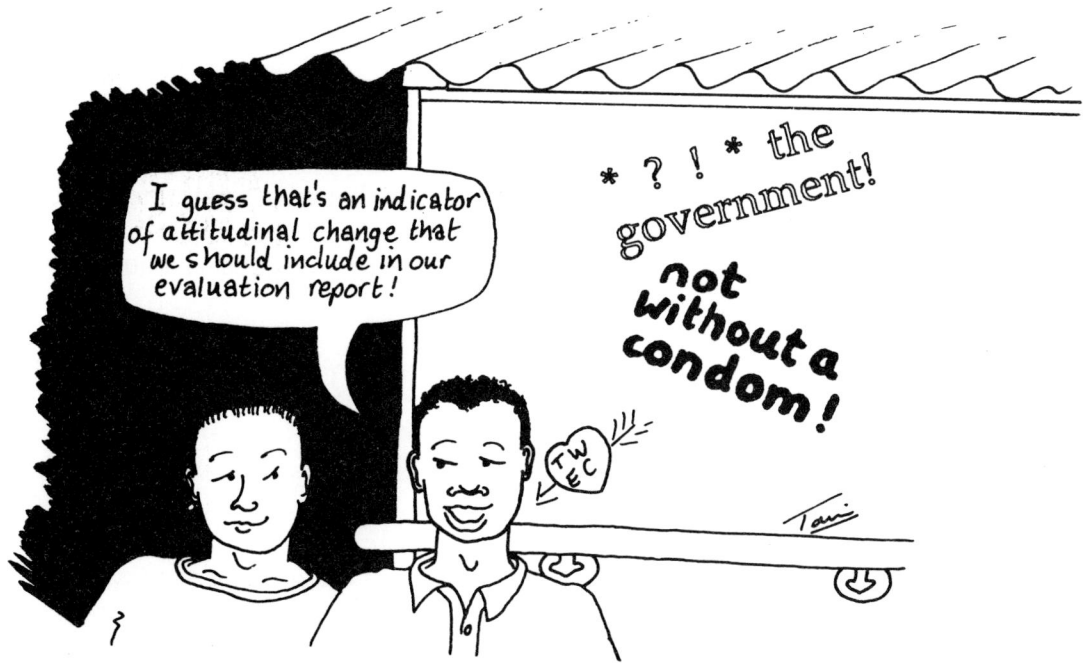

message or whether the attitudes of young people involved in an HIV/AIDS workshop have changed. For each activity, there are many questions that can be asked about its outcomes.

Knowing why an activity succeeds or fails is as important as knowing what its outcomes are. It is therefore important to ask questions about *how* an activity works, *what* made things happen and *what* support mechanisms were in place to enable progress to be made. This is usually called *process evaluation* (see page 32). Questions to be asked here include: what are the roles of the participants in the activity, who are the stakeholders (participants, managers, service providers), what are the qualities and motivation of others involved in the activity, and does the activity meet the needs of all participants? For each activity, there will be many such questions worthy of investigation.

The scope of an evaluation is likely to be determined both by the resources available and by the nature of the HIV/AIDS health promotion activity itself. While evaluation cannot be expected to do everything, it may be reasonable to expect an evaluation to achieve some or all of the following objectives:

- To identify the main achievements or failings of an HIV/AIDS health promotion activity.
- To show where and how changes need to be made.
- To show how the strengths of a particular activity can be built upon.
- To provide information for planning and decision making.
- To help those involved to see the wider context and implications of their work.(4)

Exercise 8 **What to evaluate?**

Aim To help you to decide what to evaluate.

Choose a specific project with identified aims and objectives. Brainstorm a list of possible issues that an evaluation could address. Use the following set of questions as a guide if you find it helpful:

- Why?
- What?
- When?
- Where?
- Who?
- How?

Allow plenty of time to identify a broad range of issues. Do not think too closely about specific ideas until the list is complete, since this may stifle your creativity. You can generate even more ideas by asking your colleagues to join you in identifying the options. Keep this list for use in Exercise 10.

Who evaluates?

It is often assumed that evaluation is something done by 'experts', but evaluation can be carried out either externally by experts or internally by those running/participating in the activity. There are many different reasons for choosing either external or internal evaluation.

The main advantage of external evaluators is that they will have a certain amount of expertise and time to dedicate to the evaluation, and they may also be seen to have greater credibility in the eyes of outsiders.(3) This latter factor may be important if the evaluation is to influence policy decisions. External evaluators are also able to bring an element of 'objectivity' to the evaluation, in that they are not personally involved. For example, external evaluators may be less influenced by the personal friendships, as well as by the likes and dislikes of the activity staff, and they can remain relatively unaffected by the normal power structure of the working environment. External evaluators may, however, have concerns of their own, such as the pressure to generate more research money and the need to produce publications. They will also have a variety of personal traits, beliefs and attitudes that will affect their supposedly 'objective' viewpoint. It is important therefore to recognise that even external evaluators can never be entirely neutral in the stance they take.

It is also crucially important that external evaluators understand the context of HIV/AIDS health promotion. They will need commitment and sensitivity to work in an area that often raises complex issues concerned with race, gender, class, sexuality and the rights of minority communities. HIV/AIDS health promotion evaluators therefore need a degree of broadmindedness that may not always be found in those who evaluate other types of health promotion work. Evaluators also need to be aware of the constraints that may shape the success of the activity. They should, for example, be aware of the level of managerial support, the degree of access that workers have to budgets, workers' status in relation to other employees, etc.

If the evaluation is 'imposed', this may be seen by those involved in the activity as a threatening and judgemental process, as something that attempts to apportion blame for apparent 'failures'. This may cause workers to have a low level of

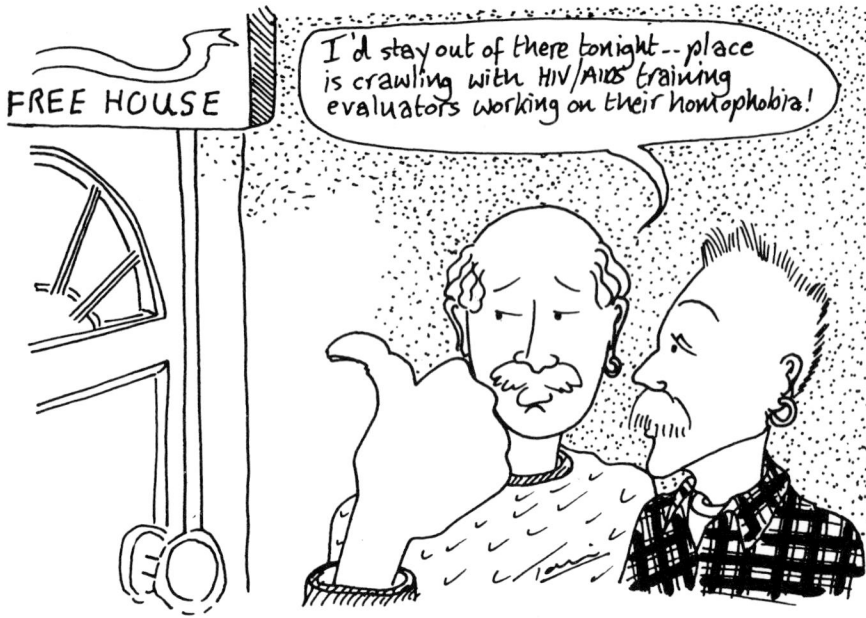

commitment to the evaluation, with the result that the evaluation may become a painful process. It may be necessary in some cases to draw up a contract with the external evaluator, by which the process of evaluation can be negotiated and agreed. Issues such as the maintenance of confidentiality and the ownership of data should be clarified at the beginning of the evaluation. It is important in such a situation that local workers are assertive and negotiate, as far as possible, their relationship with evaluators. It should be possible for both evaluators and those who are being evaluated to learn from the success, mistakes and setbacks of the evaluation in order to develop the activity further and to enhance the working environment.

With these considerations in mind, and in some situations, it may be more appropriate for internal evaluation to take place. Here, the evaluation is undertaken by a person involved in the development of the activity or by someone who knows the activity well. Such a person may know the ways in which the activity functions, and is likely to be aware of its objectives, problems, strengths and weaknesses. The person chosen is also likely to have a good understanding of the issues raised by the HIV/AIDS activity, as well as an interest in seeing that the activity is as successful as possible. An internal evaluator may not be truly 'objective', but the advantages of knowledge and sensitivity towards an activity may need to be weighed against this.

In some circumstances, the nature of the HIV/AIDS health promotion activity demands the involvement of an internal evaluator. Here, the presence of an external evaluator in the role of 'neutral observer' may be at odds with the ethos of the activity. For example, in a community-based HIV/AIDS health promotion activity, it may be entirely inappropriate for an external evaluator who has had no prior involvement in the development of the activity, and who may in some situations maintain overly static notions of success, to evaluate a dynamic and ever-changing course of events.(5) It is also important to consider the extent to which an external evaluator genuinely understands the goals of the activity.

As an alternative in such circumstances, evaluation may be best attempted by those participating in the activity. Participatory evaluation involves the people taking part in the activity deciding when and how to evaluate, selecting the methods to be used, collecting and analysing data and information, preparing reports, and deciding how to use the results and put the recommendations into practice. Participants not only evaluate what they have got out of the activity, but also what they have put into it and what it has achieved. Evaluation by the participants themselves can be a dynamic process, where those involved in the activity become responsive and adaptable throughout, and where judgemental decision making and the need to apportion blame are reduced.

These are some of the issues that need to be considered when deciding who is to evaluate. When there is a choice, it can often be tempting to opt for an external evaluation, so that the burden of evaluation can be passed to someone else. It is, however, particularly important to consider the nature and ethos of the activity, and the effect that the evaluation may have on either inhibiting or developing the activity – external evaluation may not always be the easiest or most appropriate option.

Exercise 9 **The 'good' evaluator**

Aim   To help you to identify some of the qualities that a 'good' evaluator might have.

Design a person specification for the evaluator(s) of a particular HIV/AIDS health promotion project by completing the chart on page 28. If you envisage a division of labour within an evaluation team, you may wish to formulate several person specifications.

Does the completed specification suggest who the evaluator(s) should be? Should they be service providers, participants or external experts?

Does the exercise suggest issues that need to be considered before an evaluation is arranged (e.g. prior training, extra channels for communicating and making evaluation-related decisions, additional support for affected staff and volunteers, etc.)?

Person specification for an evaluator of an HIV/AIDS health promotion project

Attributes	Essential	Desirable
Knowledge and qualifications: e.g. awareness of equal opportunity issues, knowledge of theories of adult learning, injecting drug use, etc.		
Skills: e.g. numeracy, communicating with young people, questionnaire design, report writing, etc.		
Qualities and attitudes: e.g. understanding of HIV/AIDS specific issues, being warm, accurate and methodical, etc.		
Experience: e.g. talking about sex with strangers, negotiating within a medical bureaucracy, working within a tight budget, etc.		
Other factors: e.g. access to a computer, evening work, must be known to service users, estimated deadline for completing data collection, etc.		

When to evaluate?

Ideally, evaluation should be planned alongside the development of an activity. It is important that evaluation does not become something that is 'tacked on' later. However, the decision about when to evaluate will depend on the nature and objectives of the activity. There may be several factors to consider when deciding when to evaluate. These include:

- Does the activity have long-term objectives? If it has, it will be useless trying to evaluate the outcome of the activity too soon, and it may be appropriate to evaluate some time after

the project has ended. For example, a long-term objective of a training course may be to enhance general practitioners' attitudes toward injecting drug users. This may be evaluated perhaps a year after the initial training to assess its long-term effects.
- Does the activity have short-term objectives? In this case, evaluation may take place immediately after the activity has ended. For example, a short-term objective of a training course may be that there should be a comfortable environment in which participants can relax. This can be easily evaluated during or immediately following the course.
- What kind of information is to be included in a process evaluation? Do records need to be maintained on how the activity was set up? If so, the evaluation process may begin as soon as the activity begins. Or if participants are to be actively involved in the evaluation, they may want to keep records of the activity, as well their thoughts and feelings, at the time.
- Are external evaluators to be involved in the evaluation? If so, this will affect timing. For example, the timing may be imposed, or the evaluation may be delayed while searching for appropriate evaluators.

Since the evaluation of long-term objectives and short-term objectives may need to be initiated at different times, it is essential that, wherever possible, evaluation is planned at the time the activity is being set up.

The scope of evaluation

When planning an evaluation, it is important to recognise that constraints of time and resources will limit its scope. It is necessary to consider how long the evaluation will take and how much it will cost. The time-scale of the evaluation will depend on several factors, such as how many people are involved, how many people will work on the evaluation, how long it will take to prepare relevant materials (such as questionnaires and survey forms) and how much data can be handled. It is also important to consider the cost of materials such as paper, typing, photocopying, and also the amount of effort and labour put into the evaluation that could have been spent elsewhere.

It is therefore important to set 'boundaries' or realistic limits to the scope of the evaluation. Do not expect to be able to evaluate every aspect of the activity thoroughly; rather, use the available time and resources wisely. For example, when evaluating a needle exchange scheme, it may be interesting to survey who uses the scheme, where the users travel from and how representative they are of the drug-using community. As this in itself could form the basis of a research project, it may be more feasible to design a simple reaction sheet to give out with the injecting equipment. While the response rate to such a questionnaire may be low, it could provide some useful information.

Exercise 10 Priorities for evaluation

Aim To help you to refine evaluation objectives and rank them in order of priority.

Refer back to the issues you generated in Exercise 8 (page 24). Using the mnemonic ST CRAVE (pages 18–19), assess the issues you have brainstormed. Finally, refine the remaining list of issues, needs and functions into an aim and set of objectives for an evaluation of your chosen project. If you find you have a long list of objectives, prioritise them so that you end up with no more than five key objectives on which to focus the evaluation programme. The following questions may help you to choose these:

- Who is the evaluation for and what concerns them most?
- Are those involved likely to co-operate in addressing these issues?
- Can the issue under consideration be resolved accurately, conclusively and ethically?
- Can the data necessary to address this issue be gained easily and at an affordable cost?
- How long would it take to get the necessary information to answer evaluation questions meaningfully, and is this allowed for within the time-scale?

Remember that evaluation will always take time, but the rewards it brings, such as being able to plan activities better in the future, will mean that it is rarely a waste of time. Furthermore, in an area fraught with uncertainty, evaluation may contribute to an assessment of our own effectiveness.

Conclusions

When planning an evaluation it is vital to take into account the full range of issues considered in this chapter. It is important to define clearly the reasons for the evaluation, to outline what will be

Planning evaluation 31

evaluated within the limits of time and resources, and to state when and by whom the evaluation will be carried out.

Exercise 11 **Evaluation contracts**

Aim To help you to draw up an effective contract between yourself and an evaluator.

What expectations do you have about how evaluators should do their job? Are these expectations shared by all concerned?

Draft a contract for a particular project that takes account of the following issues. Be as specific as you can, as an explicit agreement between all interested parties can protect you from much subsequent frustration and misunderstanding.

- Who is paying for the evaluation and how?
- To whom are the evaluators responsible?
- To whom do they report?
- Who is the anticipated audience for the final evaluation report?
- Are reports to be given verbally or in writing?
- Who should be consulted when planning the evaluation and when?
- What budgets are available and how are they accessed?
- What is the time-scale of the evaluation and are there any deadlines, fixed times, etc.?
- Are there any other constraints, e.g. access to key personnel, data, ethical or practical considerations such as confidentiality, known conflicts of interest, etc.?
- What will be the extent/boundaries of the task/ responsibilities?
- Who has access to the data, reports, etc.?
- Who will own the data, evaluation report, etc.?
- What support is available for the evaluators and participants?
- What channels are available for resolving grievances?

When developing an evaluation contract, you may wish to include the following:

- A statement of the aims and objectives of the activity to be evaluated (pages 18–19).
- A statement of the aims and objectives of the evaluation itself (pages 23–25).
- A person specification (pages 27–28).

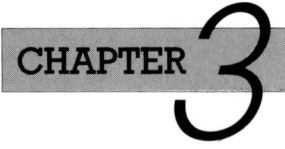

CHAPTER 3: How to evaluate – process evaluation

- Eliciting participants' views • Interviewing
- Focus group work • Reaction sheets • Diaries
- Discussion sessions • Group questionnaires
- Ad hoc techniques • Record keeping

Introduction

As we have already seen, outcome evaluation is concerned with assessing *what* an activity has achieved. Process evaluation, on the other hand, tries to explain *how* these outcomes have been brought about. Ideally, any evaluation should focus on processes as well as outcomes, as the former have a crucial effect on the latter.

Process evaluation, or formative evaluation as it is sometimes called, has a particularly important role to play in the evaluation of many local HIV/AIDS health promotion activities. It is essential for lessons to be learned from the experience of others, and for the knowledge gained to be shared and used in the development of future work. Process evaluation contributes to this by providing information on how an activity has been organised and managed. It can therefore be used to demonstrate why a particular activity has or has not been a success. Through process evaluation, issues such as the feasibility, acceptability and transferability can be examined.

There is no blueprint as to the best way to approach process evaluation.(3) The precise approach will vary with the setting and type of activity being undertaken. Process evaluation usually involves collecting a wide range of information from a variety of sources. It may involve maintaining records over a period of time to document the development of the activity, as well as the development of systematic techniques of evaluation, including interviewing, diary keeping and the use of questionnaires.

Eliciting participants' views

Process evaluation uses information from a variety of sources to gain an understanding of the range of factors that may have influenced the outcome of HIV/AIDS health promotion work. This will most certainly involve collecting information from those who participated in the activity. Participants' views can be elicited in a variety of ways. These may include interviewing, focus group work, reaction sheets, keeping diaries, and using discussion sessions and group questionnaires. It may be beneficial to use

How to evaluate – process evaluation 33

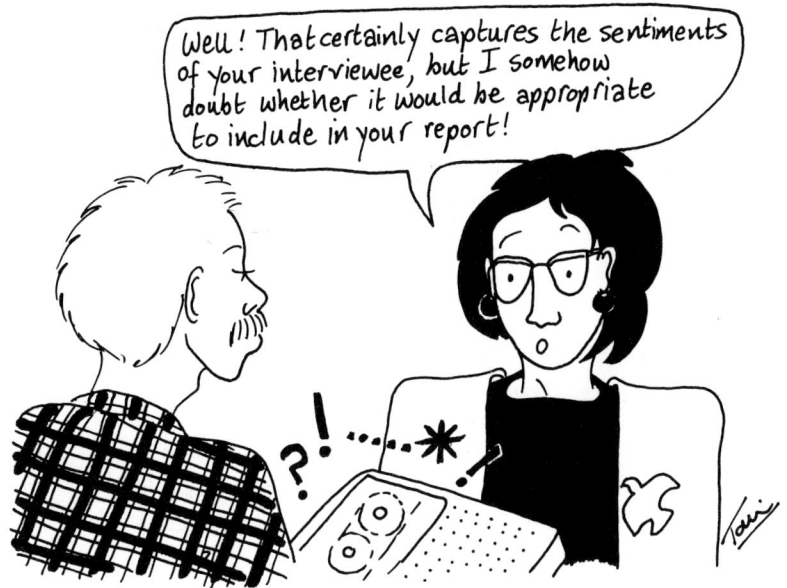

several different methods to get an 'all round view'. In this way, it may be possible not only to assess how the activity has influenced behaviour, knowledge or attitudes, but also to obtain information on such things as the relationship between facilitators and participants, the interaction between participants and the levels of communication, all of which influence the success of the activity.

Exercise 12 **Skills and qualities for effective communication**

Aim To help you to identify some of the skills that could be useful when interviewing.

The following list represents some of the personal skills, qualities and behavioural traits that are found in people who are effective interviewers and communicators. Rate yourself in the areas listed on a scale from 0 (very weak) through 5 (adequate) to 10 (very strong). This will enable you to make an initial personal assessment and to identify areas of relative weakness. Date and keep a copy of your response as you may find it helpful to repeat the exercise at a later date. You may also like to ask a colleague who knows you well to rate your strengths and weaknesses, so that you can compare your impressions with those of others.

A. *Empathy*: I try to see the world through the eyes of others; I listen well to what others say both verbally and otherwise, and I am usually able to respond. ☐

B. *Warmth and respect*: I am able to feel and show I am 'for' others; that I respect them; I can accept others even when I don't approve of things they do. ☐

C. *Genuineness*: I do not hide behind roles or facades; others know who I am and where I stand; I can say 'no' or 'I don't know' thereby establishing limits in relationships, so that my 'yes' is meaningful; I am myself in relationships. ☐

D. *Concreteness*: I am not vague when I speak to others; I deal with concrete experience, feelings and behaviour when I talk. ☐

E. *Initiative*: In relationships, I act rather than react; I reach out to contact others rather than waiting for them to contact me; I am spontaneous and can take the initiative. ☐

F. *Optimism and confidence*: Generally, I look at change and the future with confidence and hope; while not denying negative feelings and realistic worries, I like myself and relate confidently to other people. ☐

G. *Acceptance of ambiguity and uncertainty*: I appreciate that I will not always understand the complexities of a situation; I tolerate not being able to provide immediate solutions. ☐

H. *Interest and imagination*: I am curious and take an interest in the world; I enjoy being playful and imaginative. ☐

I. *Flexibility*: While I know where I stand, I am not rigid in my attitudes or behaviour; I am able to be open minded in my dealings with others and the world. ☐

J. *Verbal fluency*: I am skilled at communicating what I mean and feel. ☐

Now answer the following questions:

- What was your overall impression of the exercise? In your opinion, were any of the qualities listed *not* related to effective interviewing? Which were these?
- Did you have particular difficulties in assessing yourself in relation to any of the qualities? What conclusions might you draw from this?

- What are your three strongest and three weakest qualities?
- Will you ask some people who know you well to assess you? What factors will influence your decision?
- How could you practise and improve on those qualities that you have identified as your weakest?
- How could you build further on your areas of strength in communicating and interviewing?

Interviewing

A process evaluation may include a series of in-depth interviews with stakeholders, participants, a sample of the target audience, as well as those involved in running and organising the activity. An interview may be used to obtain information about people's reaction to or knowledge of the health promotion activity. It may aim to identify feelings towards the activity, and it may reveal stresses and strains within the activity. Interviews are also useful in revealing people's expectations about an activity and the extent to which these have been met.

When developing an interview schedule, it is important to have a clear idea of the aims of the interview and what kind of data is to be collected. Interviews can be structured or unstructured, where the choice depends to a certain extent on the aims of the interview and the skill of the interviewer.

In a structured interview, the interviewer uses a list of questions which are designed to be asked in a specific order, to try to obtain certain information. The way in which the interview is conducted and the content of the interview are worked out in advance. A structured interview is usually easier for less skilled interviewers to carry out. The data collected might also be easier to collate.

In an unstructured interview, the interviewer does not use a questionnaire or a list of preset questions but collects data in a more conversational way. The interviewer may use phrases such as 'Tell me', 'What do you think about...' or 'We are interested in...'. The interview is flexible, and the skilled interviewer will adapt the questions to the respondent's answers. The respondent's thoughts and interests will therefore guide the interview. The interviewer may follow up on particular issues by probing further to gain more information. Probing may be verbal or non-verbal, or may take the form of direct questions such as 'Please tell me more'. It is important that probing is neutral and does not suggest one particular answer to the respondent.

Structured or unstructured interviews may be used in a variety of situations. If an HIV/AIDS health promotion activity is directed at a whole community, interviews may be carried out with a sample of those involved.(5) Similarly, interviews may be carried out either with a sample of participants taking part in a series of HIV/AIDS training courses over a period of time or with all the participants involved in a particular HIV/AIDS training session.

The success of interviewing depends to a large extent on the skill of the interviewer. Often, respondents react more to their relationship with the interviewer than to the content of the questions they are actually asked. It is important therefore for the right kind of relationship between the interviewer and respondent to be established early on, especially if the interviewer is to ask personal or sensitive questions. It is particularly important for the interviewer to create a relaxed atmosphere that encourages the respondent to talk freely, and for the interviewer to be able to maintain an unbiased attitude when asking questions and recording answers.

Exercise 13 **Identifying interviewing skills**

Aim To help you to identify some of the more successful techniques for obtaining reliable and valid responses in interviews.

A. Write out a list of 'do's' and 'don'ts' to remind yourself about how to conduct unstructured interviews. Try to include at least five 'do's' and five 'don'ts'.

B. Examine the following examples and choose the interviewer response that you consider most helpful in establishing a relaxed relationship and moving matters on. For each response, identify what is helpful/unhelpful about it. Now try writing down your own response to each statement.

Example 1

Respondent: Well, really, I still feel confused about safer sex ... I've got so many unanswered questions.

Interviewer 1: Oh yes, I know what you mean. Everyone always goes on about penetrative sex as though there's nothing else anyway.

Interviewer 2: You're feeling some confusion about safer sex. Can you give me an example of a question that remains unanswered for you?

Interviewer 3: Have you got one of our leaflets? If you read it, you should understand the basic facts much more.

Example 2

Respondent: My health visitor and I just rub each other up the wrong way ... sometimes I think I'd be better off without her help.

Interviewer 1: Oh that must be so horrible for you. I really sympathise. Have you tried counting to ten when she irritates you?

Interviewer 2: Rubs you up the wrong way?

Interviewer 3: I'm sure she can't be that bad. They have really good training you know.

Example 3

Respondent: When I rang up the AIDS helpline, I felt really pleased with myself for taking the plunge and really grateful that someone listened to me.

Interviewer 1: Yeah, I've found them really helpful too. When I rang up the helpline, I just ended up crying and crying ... did that happen to you?

Interviewer 2: Oh well, that's excellent, you did really well, I really admire someone who can do things like that. I'm so pleased with you and so proud of the progress you have made since you've been coming to the centre.

Interviewer 3: It sounds like you felt you were brave and got some support. Is that how it felt?

C. Now add to your list of 'do's' and 'don'ts', if necessary.

Evaluators may not necessarily do the interviewing themselves. For example, if an HIV/AIDS health promotion activity is community based, such as providing HIV/AIDS information to Asian women in a specific community, it may be appropriate to train and to use interviewers from within that community. It is vitally important that the interviewer has an understanding of the language and the jargon that respondents use, to avoid misunderstanding, and is able to approach the situation with sensitivity.

Interviewers should try to record all the answers they are given during an interview. Trying to remember them to write them down later will lead to inaccuracy. It is important to try to record the respondent's own words in full and not paraphrase or summarise, as this may distort what was originally meant. It is sometimes a good idea to tape record an interview, although the respondent should always be aware of this and asked for permission beforehand. You will also need to be aware of the legal implications of the Data Protection Act. (Check with your local library.)

Focus group work

Focus group interviews are a way of obtaining information about the feelings and opinions of a small group of participants. They involve bringing together, usually for a single session lasting an hour or so, a group of people who have participated in the activity under review, or an appropriate representative sample. In a discussion facilitated by a competent, sensitive group worker, the group is encouraged to explore and express views on a range of predetermined topics and questions.(6)

The facilitator takes a key role in a focus group interview by creating a situation where all participants feel relaxed and are able to share their views. The facilitator will prompt and seek to clarify the participants' views by asking questions such as 'Why is that?', 'You feel that way because . . . ?' and 'Can you explain that further?' To obtain useful information, the atmosphere must be conducive to freedom of expression and each person's views must be seen to be respected. It is likely that the members of the group will not be homogeneous, so the facilitator must be able to deal with variations in skills and experience, as well as any inequalities of power that exist between participants.

Data from focus group work can be analysed in different ways depending on the purpose of the interview. The session may be taped, from which notes can be made and the general findings reported. Alternatively, a full and accurate transcript may be made of the tapes, from which a list of key ideas, words and phrases can be generated, including verbatim quotes that capture sentiments. Categories of concern can then be defined by clustering similar ideas and quotes together. From this, the most pertinent themes and trends can be identified.

Reaction sheets

Reaction sheets are a simple kind of questionnaire that asks questions about people's satisfaction with a particular activity. They are a popular evaluation technique because they are easy

How to evaluate – process evaluation 39

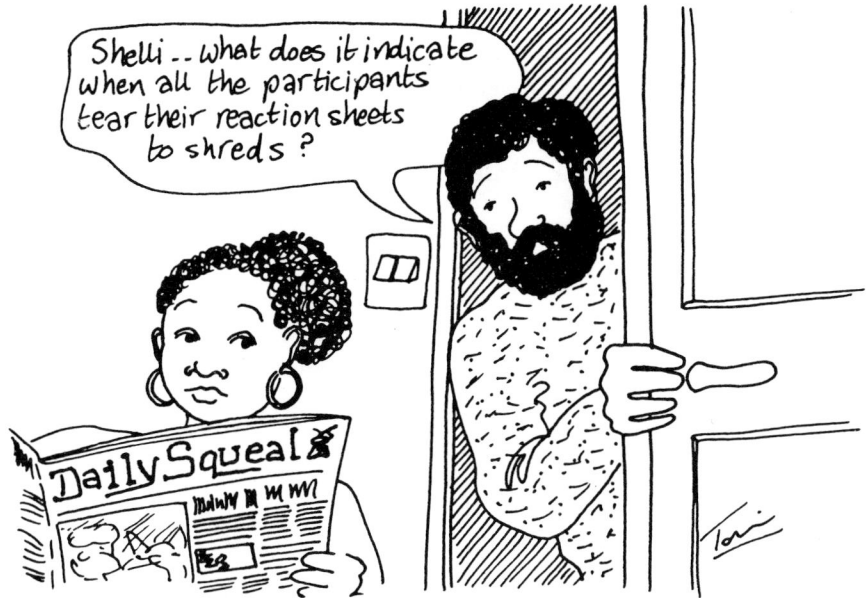

to administer. There are, however, several things to watch out for when using reaction sheets.

First, people often give favourable responses to a health promotion activity, so a large number of positive responses does not necessarily indicate that the activity has been a success. On the other hand, if there is a large number of negative responses, this should be seen as an indication for change.

Second, general questions such as 'Did you enjoy the activity?' are likely to generate favourable but inaccurate answers. More specific questions such as 'Did the trainer answer all your questions about HIV transmission?' may encourage more accurate and honest responses. It is likely that if the training course was a day or more in length, participants will have found only part of it useful or enjoyable. It might therefore be more useful to ask questions about each section of the course, to gain a more sensitive picture of what went on.

Third, individuals with different backgrounds and knowledge may assess an activity using different criteria and standards of worth. A good reaction sheet should try to reflect this.

Finally, a reaction sheet should clearly relate to the nature of the activity. If, for example, the training is of a participatory style, the emphasis of the reaction sheet should be as much on what the participants put into the activity as on what the trainer or facilitator provided. Such a reaction sheet might include questions such as 'What did you contribute to the session?', 'What did you gain from the activity?', 'Did you feel comfortable taking part in the exercises?' and 'What could you have done to make yourself or others more comfortable?'. In this way, participants can be encouraged to acknowledge responsibility for the part they played in the training.

Exercise 14 Reaction sheets

Aim To provide guidance on how to prepare a reaction sheet.

Imagine you are running a series of training workshops to increase local workers' awareness, knowledge and sensitivity towards HIV-related issues. The aim of one particular session is to increase people's ability to support individuals who may be directly affected by HIV. You decide to carry out a process evaluation of this session, gathering information through reaction sheets to be completed by all participants at the end.

In the session, people watch 'trigger scenes' on a video, where four individuals, in turn, make brief comments about HIV. The video is stopped after each scene and participants are asked to write down their 'gut reactions' and how they would respond to this person. Afterwards, they discuss their responses in pairs, which is followed by a group discussion of feelings, attitudes and effective responses. The four trigger comments are as follows:

> I know my son's got AIDS or if he hasn't yet he soon will 'cos he's been using drugs.

> When I told my girlfriend I'd tested negative, she said it made no difference – she didn't love me any more.

> Peter is furious I've told my sister he has HIV – says that I've betrayed him. He just doesn't see it is difficult for me to cope with the thought that our baby might die from AIDS.

> What gets me is that they didn't even ask if it was true. They just withdrew from the sale. Must have believed HIV can lurk in the ruddy brickwork or something!

Design a reaction sheet that will help you to find out about the following:

- What participants thought of the exercise.
- What, if anything, participants learned from taking part in the workshop.
- Which of the following factors affected their learning: how the task was structured, their individual personalities, and how and by whom the session was run.

How could you assess the design of your reaction sheet?

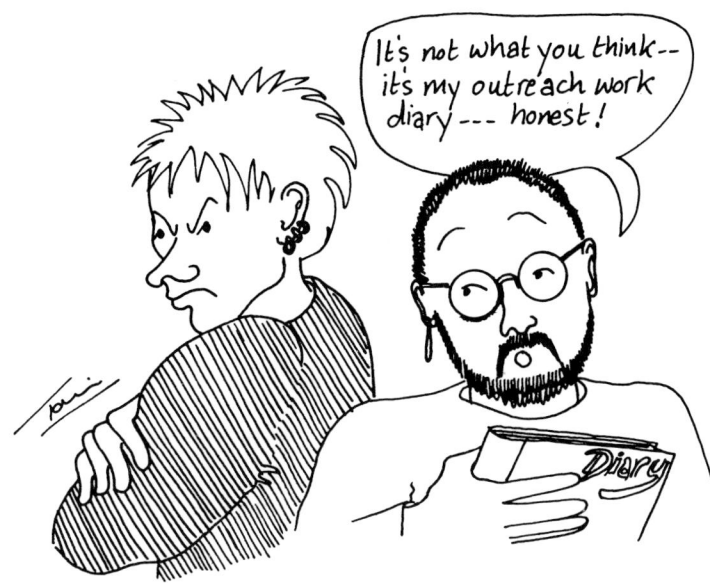

Diaries

If the same participants are involved in an activity over a period of time, such as in a series of HIV/AIDS training sessions, it may be feasible for them to keep a diary of their thoughts and feelings about the activity. This diary can be written up during or after each session, and the participants may be invited to make notes on how they feel, what they have learned, what they liked or disliked, and what was most difficult for them. In this way, a record can be kept of the progress of the activity over time. At the end of the activity, participants may like to discuss their diaries as a group, or it may be possible to produce a group diary from entries in the individual diaries. It is also important for the leaders and facilitators of the activity to keep their own diaries.

Discussion sessions

Tape recording a discussion session during, for example, an HIV/AIDS training course may provide interesting information not only about knowledge and attitudes towards HIV/AIDS, but also about the interaction between participants and facilitators, and between the participants themselves. It can be particularly useful to tape record a discussion session at the beginning and at the end of an activity to help to assess any changes that have occurred and the ways in which things have developed. It is important when using tape recordings to ensure that confidentiality is respected at all times. This may involve keeping tapes, notes and transcripts securely locked away and, when using quotations in a written report, ensuring that the individuals concerned have given permission for their remarks to be cited. All participants should consent to the use of the tape and have knowledge of what the recording will be used for. In some situations, the tape recorder may inhibit discussion, while in others it may focus the attention of the participants on the issues to be discussed. Flexibility is therefore important.

Group questionnaires

Following an activity such as a training session, a group questionnaire may be used. A group questionnaire may be similar to a self-completed questionnaire, except that small groups of four or five people discuss the questions. This may lead to a more reflective kind of evaluation with individuals identifying problems and voicing anxieties, as well as commenting on successes. Each group then reports back to the main group and a record is kept of comments made.

Ad hoc techniques

It is important in process evaluation to obtain as much information as possible in a variety of ways. *Ad hoc* evaluation techniques are limited in themselves but they may provide information that is useful to the evaluation as a whole. These techniques include 'rounds' at the end of a session, in which all participants are asked individually to say what they have most enjoyed or learned during the activity. Alternatively, participants may be asked during a session 'How do you feel at this moment?' This can give the trainer some indication of how things are going. These are techniques that many trainers use anyway to assess whether their training is on target, and they are perfectly valid techniques to use in the context of process evaluation.

Record keeping

An important aspect of process evaluation involves validating the views of participants. It is also important to know something about the history of a particular activity, as well as the social and political factors that led up to it. This kind of evaluation necessitates keeping records of the progress of the activity. This may involve an examination of relevant documents and records, discussion with key individuals and attendance at meetings. Such an assessment may reveal constraints and tensions that have affected the outcome of the activity. It may also identify the more positive interactions that have contributed to the activity's success.

Records may also be kept as a part of the process evaluation of work in progress. For example, daily logs could be kept of contacts made, lists of participants and their relevant backgrounds, resources available and resources used, extent of media coverage, number of enquiries made, requests for information, and the level of response to invitations and advertising. Although much of this information can be recorded as a matter of routine, it may be appropriate to develop a clear and concise recording system, so that such information is readily available.

Exercise 15 **Record keeping**

Aim To help you to examine the role of record keeping in your work.

- What records do you keep of your HIV/AIDS health promotion work?
- What form do these records take?
- Which are relevant to outcome evaluation and which to process evaluation?
- What are the strengths of the system you use?
- What are its weaknesses?
- Are there aspects of your work that are not recorded but could be quite easily? For instance, do you make any notes about supervision sessions? Do you enter visitors' appointments in an office diary which can be ticked, or marked 'postponed' or 'not available'?
- How can your records be used to evaluate the 'success' of your activities?
- How can you improve or consolidate your existing record systems?

A popular type of record keeping often used in outreach or community-based HIV/AIDS health promotion is fieldwork recording. For example, in an HIV/AIDS outreach project with sex workers, the outreach worker may keep detailed records of contacts made, the location of the contacts, the number of condoms given out, matters discussed, clients' comments and any referrals made. In such a way, a precise record can be kept of work in progress. This can then be used at a later date as the basis of a report. Confidentiality should be maintained at all times when keeping records,

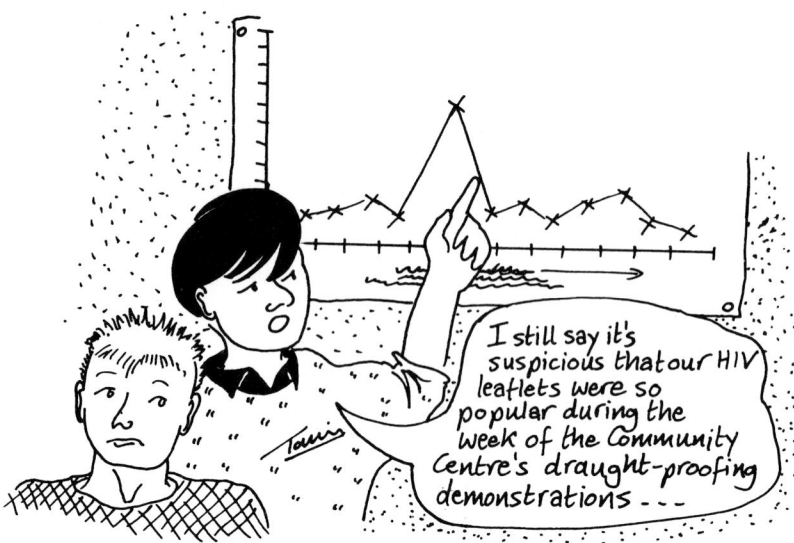

and HIV/AIDS health promoters should develop a coding system that ensures that no respondent can be traced.

Conclusions

It is clear that the evaluation of HIV/AIDS health promotion activities requires more than a simple consideration of outcomes. It also requires a consideration of the processes involved in bringing these about. Process evaluation is a means by which changes, developments, problems and issues surrounding an activity can be examined. Process evaluation also provides an opportunity to assess and to validate participants' views. It therefore plays a fundamental role in the continuing development of HIV/AIDS health promotion activities.

Although it is often implied that outcome and process evaluation offer alternative strategies, this is not the case. Ideally, most evaluations will involve both process and outcome evaluation. The emphasis given to each will depend on factors such as the nature of the activity, available resources and time, and the demands made by managers. Once a range of material has been collected, the next stage is to analyse and interpret it, an issue that is examined in more detail in Chapter 5.

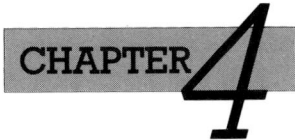

CHAPTER 4: How to evaluate – outcome evaluation

- **Indicators** • **Research designs** • **Experimental designs**
- **Surveys** • **Sampling** • **Response rates and 'drop-outs'**
- **Value for money**

Introduction

Outcome evaluation, or summative evaluation as it is sometimes called, is concerned with assessing *what* an activity has achieved. This may involve trying to assess the effectiveness of the activity by measuring changes in knowledge, attitudes or reported practices and behaviour, or by measuring outputs such as the number of people reached or the quantity of resources produced.

In assessing outcomes, two basic questions need to be addressed: namely, can a change be observed and can this change be attributed to the activity? To answer these questions, it is necessary to have a well-designed evaluation and to specify in advance an appropriate range of outcome measures or indicators of success.

Indicators

Defining appropriate indicators is an essential step in the evaluation of HIV/AIDS health promotion activities. Indicators are things that help us to identify when change has taken place. Some health promotion evaluations have attempted to measure the outcome of an activity on the basis of the changing incidence of infection, morbidity and mortality. It is unlikely, however, that a direct link can ever be drawn between a health promotion activity and subsequent changes in the incidence of disease. It is therefore necessary to identify those key factors that may influence change in the long term but can be measured more immediately. These include measures of behaviour, knowledge and attitudes, measures of input into the activity or measures of changes in social policy. Table 1 shows some of the indicators that can be used in the evaluation of HIV/AIDS health promotion work.

Three main types of indicators can be distinguished: *outcome indicators*, *intermediate indicators* and *indirect indicators*. Usually, the ultimate outcome indicator in an HIV/AIDS health promotion activity is a health status indicator that measures the incidence of HIV infection, but it is unlikely that this will be able to be used as a valid indicator in most cases. More valid outcome

Table 1 *Indicators that can be used in evaluating HIV/AIDS health promotion activities*

Type of indicator	Example
Outcome indicators	
Health status indicators	Incidence of HIV infection
Behavioural measures	Reported safer sex practice
	Reported injecting behaviour
	Reduction in risk taking
Attitude/knowledge measures	Knowledge of HIV transmission
	Knowledge about risky behaviour
	Attitude towards people with HIV
Self-concept measures	Extent of empowerment in relation to negotiation of safer sex
	Confidence in talking about safer sex
	Values and beliefs about sexuality
	Measures of self-esteem
Intermediate indicators	
Quantitative indicators	Number and type of calls received
	Number of needles and syringes exchanged
	Number of condoms distributed
Indirect indicators	
Output indicators	Number of materials produced
	Number of training sessions run
	Number of staff trained
Input indicators	Amount of human and financial resources devoted to the activity
Health/social policy indicators	Extent of workplace policies
	Extent of legislation in relation to non-discrimination
Process indicators	Extent of involvement of group members
	Relationship between participants

indicators include measures of changes in behaviour (such as the use of needle and syringe exchange schemes), measures of changes in attitudes (such as attitudes towards people with HIV) and measures of changes in knowledge (such as knowledge of how HIV is and is not transmitted).

In some situations, it may not be possible to measure changes in behaviour or knowledge directly. Here, intermediate indicators may be needed. For example, when evaluating a needle exchange scheme, it may not be possible to measure directly changes in injecting behaviour, but by recording the number of needles and syringes exchanged, it may be possible to gain some insight into what is going on.

In other circumstances, it may prove impractical to collect data on certain intermediate indicators, so more indirect measures of success may be appropriate. These may include output measures such as the number of leaflets dispensed, the number of staff trained or the number of lectures given. Further indirect measures of success include health and social policy indicators, which measure the extent to which appropriate workplace policies to prevent discrimination against people with AIDS and HIV infection have come into being, and process indicators, which assess the extent of involvement of group members in the activity, the participation of interested agencies, and the relationship and roles of group participants.

Indicators are rarely used in isolation from one another. Indirect measures and intermediate measures, for example, may be used in tandem to give an indication of a successful outcome of an HIV/AIDS activity. The choice of indicators will depend on the objectives of the activity, as well as on an understanding of the relationship between factors influencing behaviour and health status. For example, if the activity assumes that knowledge is likely to lead to a change in attitude, which is in turn likely to lead to a change in reported practices and behaviour, then data should be collected on each of these variables. If, on the other hand, the model of health promotion being used is more sophisticated, then data may be collected on other indicators as well.(7, 8) These may include measures of an individual's values, drives, self-esteem, self-concept and beliefs. Once specific indicators have been identified, the next step is to design the evaluation.

Research designs in evaluation

There are no simple rules about the best way to carry out an outcome evaluation, although several key principles need to be borne in mind no matter which approach is adopted. Two basic techniques can be used in evaluating the outcomes of HIV/AIDS health promotion – experimental designs and survey work.

Experimental designs

Outcome evaluation is very much concerned with looking at the success of an activity. It attempts to assess whether an activity has worked and what it has achieved. The crucial question that is being asked is 'Would the same or better results be achieved by doing something different, or even nothing at all?' To answer this

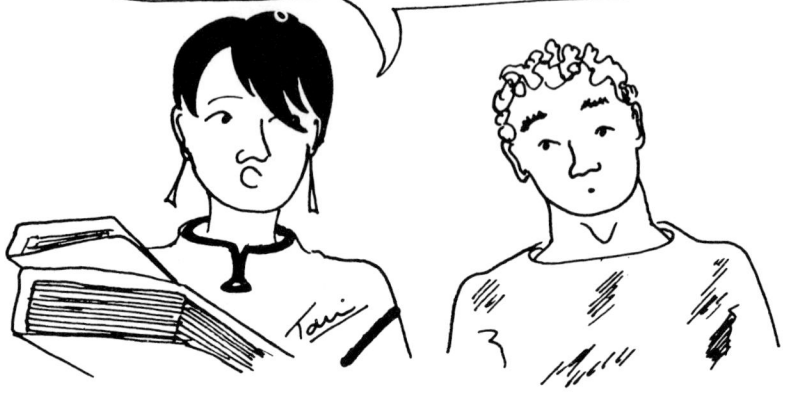

question, the evaluator has to show that any success or observed outcomes are attributable to the activity itself. To do this, the evaluator has to be able to rule out the possibility of outside influences contributing to the success (or even failure) of the activity. External factors may greatly influence the outcomes of a local activity. A national information campaign, for example, may coincide with the activity, as may sensationalist reports on television or in the tabloid press. Experimental designs attempt to give the evaluator a degree of control over such outside influences, so that the impact of the activity alone can be assessed.

In the simplest experimental design, one group of people takes part in the activity while another group does not. The group that takes part in the activity is usually called the *experimental group*, whereas the group that does not is called the *control group*. The success of the activity can then be assessed by comparing the outcomes of the experimental group against those of the control group. To ensure that there are no systematic differences between the groups that could affect the outcome, allocation to the experimental and control groups is usually done randomly.

Suppose, for example, that the aim of an evaluation is to assess student nurses' knowledge of HIV/AIDS after a two-hour HIV/AIDS training session. A list of all the nurses would be made and each one allocated a number. The nurses would then be randomly allocated to the control group or the experimental group by picking numbers out of a hat or by using special tables of random numbers.(9, 10) Those in the control group would then

Table 2 *Experimental design, post-test only, with random allocation to the two groups*

Group	Activity	Post-test
Experimental	HIV/AIDS training session	HIV/AIDS questionnaire
Control	Usual training session	HIV/AIDS questionnaire

undergo the HIV/AIDS training while those in the experimental group would undergo some other training. Measures would then be taken of each group's knowledge of HIV/AIDS (by, for example, using a questionnaire, or by setting a test) and a comparison of the results made (Table 2).

In HIV/AIDS health promotion, it is important to consider the ethics involved in the use of control groups. In some situations, for example, it would be completely inappropriate to use control groups if this meant withholding a service from those desiring it (e.g. withholding clean needles and syringes from injecting drug users). Moreover, on some occasions, the evaluator may have little direct control over who takes part in an activity. If this is the case, it may be necessary to use a *comparison group* instead of a control group. A comparison group is a group of people that resembles those taking part in the activity with respect to age, sex, social status and occupation. The difference between a control group and a comparison group is that the subjects have not been randomly assigned to the group. This means that there might be some bias: there may be important reasons why one group is taking part in the activity and another is not, which will affect the results. Those people in the experimental group, for example, may have actively sought information on HIV/AIDS, while those in the comparison group may have no particular interest in HIV/AIDS issues. To minimise any bias, a pre-test can be used to assess any initial differences between the experimental group and the comparison group, and a post-test can be used to examine any changes in these differences. For example, it would be possible to evaluate the effects of a film depicting the life of people with HIV/AIDS or the attitudes of young people towards people with HIV/AIDS by comparing the attitudes of the group of young people seeing the film with a group of young people who did not. This could be done by means of before-and-after questionnaires or interviews. The two groups would need to be matched in terms of age, sex, length of schooling, educational attainment, social background and ethnic background (Table 3).

Table 3 *Before-and-after design with a comparison group: subjects are not randomly allocated*

Group	Pre-test	Activity	Post-test
Experimental	X	X	X
Comparison	X	–	X

When it is not possible to find a suitable comparison group, the group involved in the activity can be used as its own control group by taking the same measurements at intervals before and after the activity. Here, the success of the activity is measured by assessing a trend over a period of time before and after the activity is implemented – this is called a *single group time series design*. This provides a long-term view of the effect of the activity rather than a 'snapshot'. Such an approach might be used to evaluate the effectiveness of a local campaign publicising the existence of an AIDS helpline, by comparing the number and type of calls received over a period of months before the campaign with those received following the campaign (see figure opposite).

Because of scarce resources and a shortage of time, many evaluations are based on pre- and post-tests of a single group. Unfortunately, this is the weakest possible choice of experimental design because it is not possible to ask the question 'What would happen without the activity?'. If this is the only option, however,

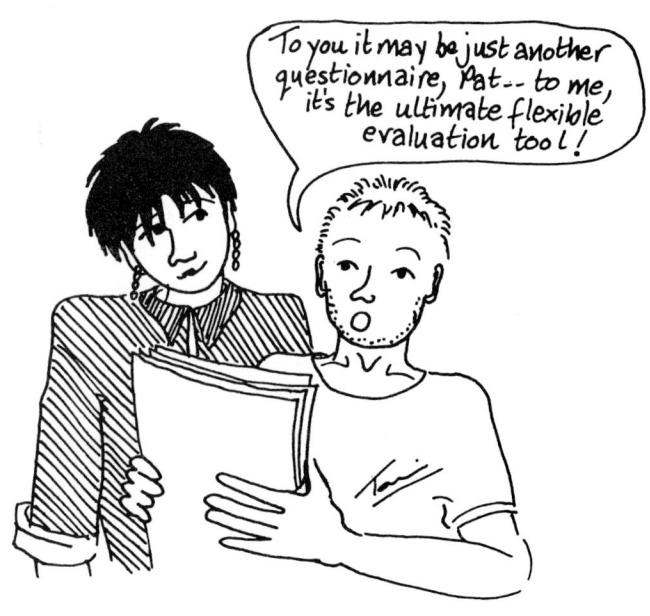

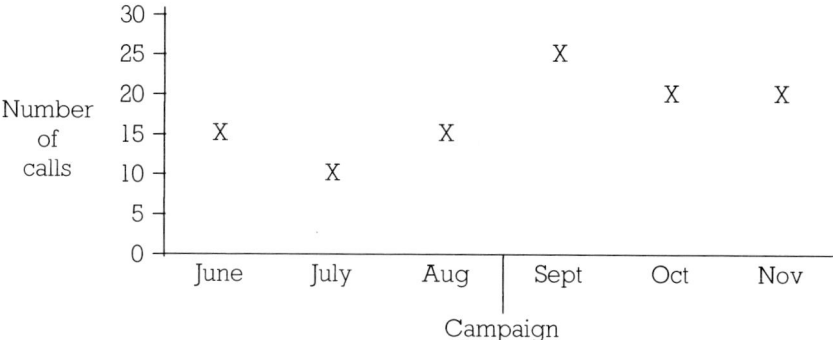

Single group time series design: number of calls to AIDS helpline before and after a publicity campaign.

the results of the evaluation can be strengthened by supplementing them with a detailed description of the programme and how it has been implemented, supported by a well-argued theoretical justification of the approach used and how this might be expected to produce the observed results.

Exercise 16 **Experimental design – single group time series**

Aim To look at the evaluation of a particular project and to consider whether the conclusions drawn are appropriate.

You have been asked to plan, run and evaluate a month-long publicity campaign for a local AIDS helpline. You produce some posters and shop window cards for display in clubs, chemists and newsagents. You also organise a series of talks, which are then reported in the local paper. Information about the helpline is included in the talks and in the articles, and you remind people that the telephone number for the AIDS helpline is in the local telephone book. In terms of evaluation, the project monitors the number and types of calls via a log sheet. You choose the single group time series approach and find that calls for the two months following the campaign are 175% higher than in the half-year preceding the campaign while calls for the next six months are 66% higher.

A. Construct a table and sketch a graph to illustrate these results.

You present a report to the management committee of the helpline and, in the discussion that follows, one committee member claims that the campaign was a waste of resources. He insists that the rise in the number of calls is due more to the anxieties raised by a frontpage article in a national tabloid, rather than to the publicity campaign. The headline proclaimed: 'Dog fleas carry AIDS'.

B. Answer the following questions:
- What factors might you cite in support of your belief that your campaign did have a significant impact?
- What evidence might you now be able to find to assess the relative impact of the tabloid feature and your publicity campaign?
- How else, with very limited resources, could you have carried out your evaluation so as to avoid this difficulty?

Surveys

Surveys are a popular way of collecting information from people about their knowledge and attitudes towards HIV/AIDS, and also about their reported behaviour and practices. Two kinds of surveys are possible – those involving *interviews* and those involving *questionnaires* (see Chapter 3). Interviews involve face-to-face data collection and vary from those that are highly structured to those that adopt a more open-ended approach. Interview data is often tape recorded, although sometimes the interviewer may keep a written record of what is said. Questionnaires, on the other hand, involve people writing down their answers to the questions asked. Once completed, questionnaires can be collected up by the evaluator or returned by post. As with interviews, both open-ended and closed questions can be asked.(11, 12)

Surveys are not as useful as experiments when it comes to identifying the cause of a particular outcome. They cannot prove that the activity itself *caused* an observed change; they can only *imply* that this is due to the activity. However, in most cases, this can be backed up by an explanation of how a particular intervention might be expected to produce the observed results.

Surveys are often used to examine the relationship between a health promotion activity and its outcomes in situations where the use of an experiment is not feasible. They usually attempt to measure the extent to which the objectives of an activity have been reached. For example, the short-term objectives of a training activity may be to increase knowledge about HIV transmission, and this can be assessed with a knowledge-based questionnaire. Activities may also have long-term objectives, such as changing the attitudes of general practitioners towards drug users, or changing the work practices of those who care for people with AIDS. This may be assessed by interviewing or administering questionnaires to participants, as well as to the people with whom they work. A well-designed survey may also reveal some of the unintended outcomes of an activity (see page 13).

As before, more knowledge about the outcome of an activity can be gained if data are collected before and after the activity is implemented. Pre- and post-activity interviews or questionnaires, for example, can assess the impact of an activity by comparing levels of knowledge or attitudes before an activity with levels of knowledge or attitudes afterwards. In a pre- and post-activity survey design, the same questionnaire or interview schedule must be used each time. In such cases, pre- and post-activity questionnaires must be presented on separate sheets to prevent respondents from being influenced by their original answers. It may also be useful to use pre-coded questions, so that an easy comparison can be made between the results.

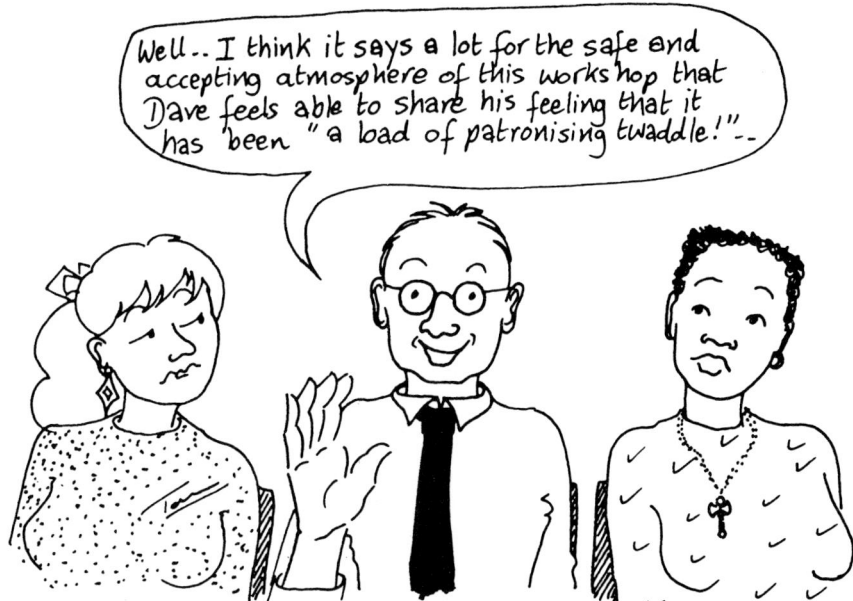

Questionnaires can sometimes be limited in their ability to elicit respondents' real attitudes and feelings. In some situations, for example, respondents may give 'correct' or acceptable answers that may not truly reflect their attitudes. For example, a questionnaire may not necessarily be able to elicit prejudice if the respondent wants to hide it. In situations like this, it may be more valid to carry out an interview, where there may be more opportunity for more in-depth enquiry.

Sampling

When evaluating training activities, it is usual for questionnaires or reaction sheets to be completed by all participants. However, when evaluating a community-based HIV/AIDS health promotion project, this may not be feasible. Here, it is unlikely that everyone in a chosen population can be surveyed, so it will be necessary to use a *sample*.

Sampling consists of choosing a small number of people from a larger group to participate in a study. The aim is to ensure that this small group is representative of the larger one. Individuals can be selected either on a probability basis or on a random basis (where each person has the same chance of being selected), or on a non-probability basis. Non-probability samples are often used when there is no complete record of who is in the group as a whole. Different kinds of non-probability samples include: *purposive sampling*, where selected individual respondents are chosen on the basis that they are 'typical' of the target group; *opportunistic sampling*, where the survey involves simply accessing all the members of the chosen group that can be reached; and *snowball sampling*, where individuals are asked to suggest other people like themselves who might take part in the survey. This last kind of non-probability sampling can be used, for example, in a local survey of the effects of an HIV/AIDS health promotion activity on the attitudes and behaviours of injecting drug users. In the case of this group, no complete list of those who could be included in the study exists and, as a result, the most convenient way of reaching possible respondents is through an existing network of contacts.

Response rates and 'drop-outs'

It is rarely possible to obtain a response from all those selected in a sample. The response rate – that is, the number of people who agree to participate in interviews or who complete and return a questionnaire – will depend on a number of factors. These include literacy, the length of time it takes to complete an interview or questionnaire, the interest it holds for respondents, the degree of anonymity offered and the use to which the data will be put. As a rule, questionnaires sent through the post will always produce a lower response than those distributed personally. These in turn will achieve a lower response rate than face-to-face interviews. It is always wise to state an explicit deadline date for the return of postal questionnaires and to send a written reminder to respondents as the date approaches. If the sample is relatively

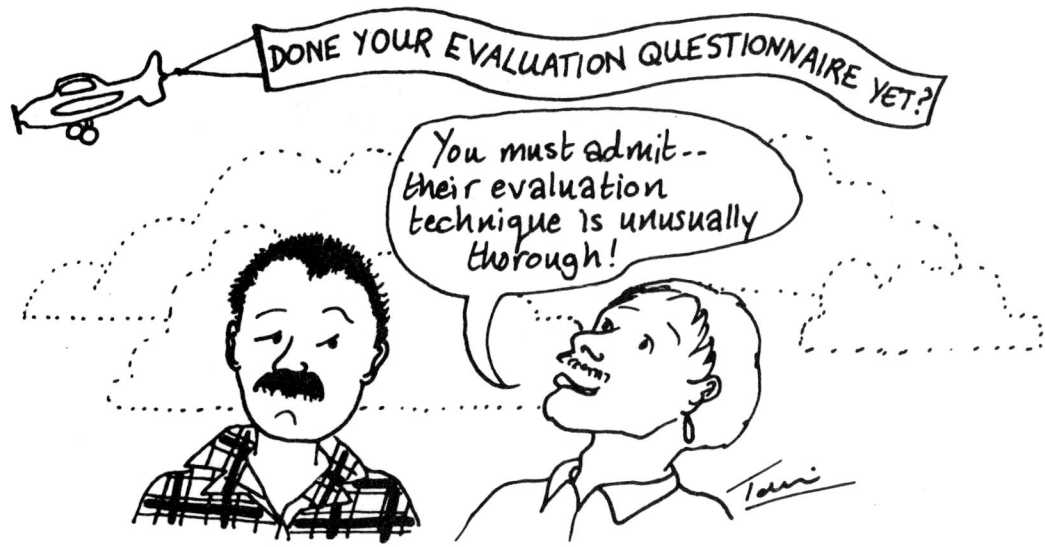

small, it can sometimes be useful to follow up the reminder with a telephone call.

Non-response can be a source of bias as non-respondents may differ from respondents in their characteristics. It is useful to maintain a record of the non-responses, and to try to distinguish between those who refuse to answer and those who fail to answer (e.g. for reasons such as being on holiday, being ill or out of the office), as this may provide some important information.

When an activity stretches over a period of time (e.g. a series of HIV/AIDS workshops), some participants may 'drop out'. It is still useful, however, to include them in the evaluation, as there may be important reasons why this happened, which may have a bearing on the future development of the activity. Drop-out may occasionally be the result of the evaluation process itself, perhaps due to its lack of sensitivity.

Value for money

When discussing measures of outcomes, it is important to consider outcomes in economic terms. All HIV/AIDS health promotion activities must take cost into account, since they all consume finite resources. There is therefore increasing pressure for evaluation to show the 'cost effectiveness' or 'cost–benefit' of HIV/AIDS health promotion activities.

There are three main ways of calculating value for money (13):

1. Cost analysis – this indicates the financial costs of competing activities.

2. Cost-effectiveness analysis – this compares the relative effectiveness of an activity (how well an activity has done) with other actual or potential activities, by identifying the relative financial costs.
3. Cost–benefit analysis – this states the financial costs and also attempts to place a price on the benefits accruing from the activity. A calculation of the cost per given benefit is then possible. This is often expressed as a cost–benefit ratio.

Cost–benefit analysis attempts to put a monetary value on as many of the costs and benefits arising from the activity as possible. However, this kind of analysis faces very real problems when it comes to placing monetary value on costs such as opportunity costs, time, labour and use of resources, and on benefits such as economic benefits, as well as improved health, reduction in pain and suffering, quality of life and increase in working life.

A complete cost–benefit analysis would also have to include an assessment of the qualitative benefits of a health promotion activity, with the weight attached to each being at the discretion of the evaluator. Cost–benefit analysis does not intrinsically assume that reducing the incidence of HIV infection is a worthwhile activity in every case. It therefore compares the financial cost of delivering the activity against the financial costs of the benefits resulting from a reduction in the incidence of HIV infection. Such an approach could be viewed as attaching a 'price' to people's lives and health, and many people question the fundamental morality of such an analysis.

Cost–benefit analysis may, however, provide useful information to help with decision making in the face of restricted resources, and it is sometimes useful for health promoters to be able to point out the relatively high cost of caring for people with HIV/AIDS compared with prevention activities. However, health promotion workers need to be cautious when making claims about saving relative health care costs. As has been discussed, it is unlikely that a direct causal link can be made between any one health promotion activity and the subsequent incidence of HIV. The 'benefits' or outcomes of the activity should therefore be measured in a way that is consistent with the objectives of the activity. For example, a health promotion activity that is designed to disseminate information about HIV transmission, or to influence health-related behaviour, should measure outcomes that reflect these objectives. This is unlikely to include immediate or measurable improvements in the rate of incidence of HIV infection.

Cost-effectiveness analysis does not require expressing the outputs of an activity in monetary terms; therefore, it avoids the problem of assigning monetary value to qualitative outcomes. Monetary value is not assigned in cost-effectiveness analysis, since it is concerned only with choosing between two alternatives. The chosen alternative is described as being the most cost-effective way of changing, for example, knowledge, attitude and behaviour. The value of cost-effectiveness analysis of outcomes lies in its ability to ensure that particular outcomes are brought about in the most effective way. For example, the setting up of a pharmacy-based needle exchange scheme may be compared with general practitioners providing routine advice and clean injecting equipment. The effectiveness of each activity would be shown by indicators such as the number of needles and syringes exchanged, the number of clients using the service, the amount of time and resources devoted to each client, and the comparative costs.

Exercise 17 **Costs and cost effectiveness**

Aim To provide you with an opportunity to examine critically a project in relation to its cost.

Imagine the publicity campaign evaluated in Exercise 16 cost £2183.

Volunteer expenses (lunch and travel for 4 volunteers for 24 days @ £6/day)	576
Poster: designs	200
Poster: printing (500 copies)	805
Stationery	147
Hospitality	38
Photocopying	166
Postage	62
Hire of training venues (£15 × 4)	60
Shop window ads (43 ads for 12 weeks at 25p/week)	129
	£2183

If you were asked to report on cost, costs–benefits and cost effectiveness, what main points might you make in relation to each of the expenditure headings?

Conclusions

Outcome evaluation is concerned with assessing what an activity has achieved. To do this, it is important to adopt a rigorous approach that can clearly demonstrate what has been achieved and how that achievement can be related to the interventions that have taken place.

When evaluating the outcomes of HIV/AIDS health promotion, it is important to ensure that unchallenged beliefs and overly ambitious expectations of what an activity can achieve do not cause an evaluation to focus on inappropriate outcomes. For example, it is pointless to examine changes in behaviour when an activity could only realistically be expected to disseminate information about the nature of HIV transmission and associated health risks.

In some respects, and if used uncritically, outcome evaluation may adopt too simplistic an 'input–output' approach, by suggesting that the effects of an HIV/AIDS health promotion activity can easily be identified and evaluated. It is important that these issues are borne in mind when carrying out outcome evaluation.

CHAPTER 5: Producing evaluation reports

- **Analysing information** • **Interpreting results**
- **Writing reports**

Introduction

Any evaluation of HIV/AIDS work will produce a large amount of both qualitative and quantitative information. This needs to be collated and analysed in a way that shows the findings of the evaluation clearly and precisely, as well as any recommendations that may arise. When analysing data and writing evaluation reports, several key principles should be borne in mind.

Analysing information

Analysing the information collected involves processing it to reveal patterns or themes. This may be achieved, for example, by calculating the average score on a knowledge test, or the percentage of people 'enjoying' an activity. Alternatively, it may include reviewing and classifying qualitative data in a meaningful way.

The first step in analysis is to assemble all the information collected by an evaluation and to set it out so that any emerging trends can be identified. This will involve the use of several different techniques if the evaluation includes both quantitative

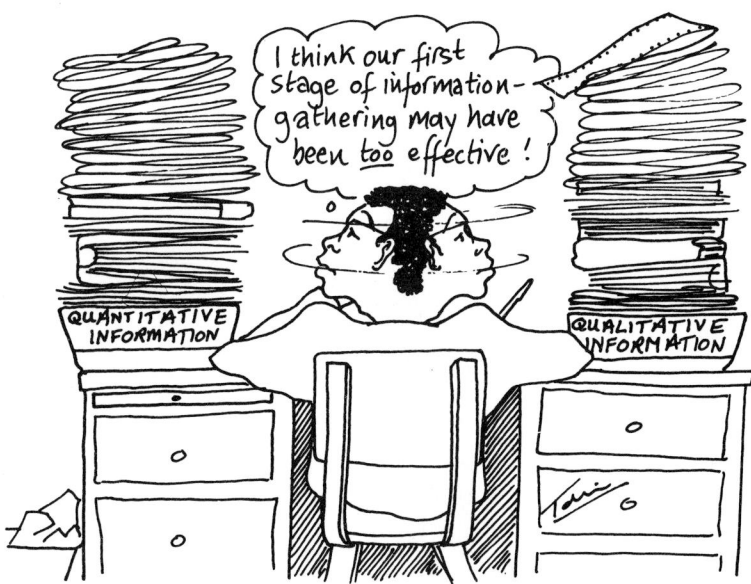

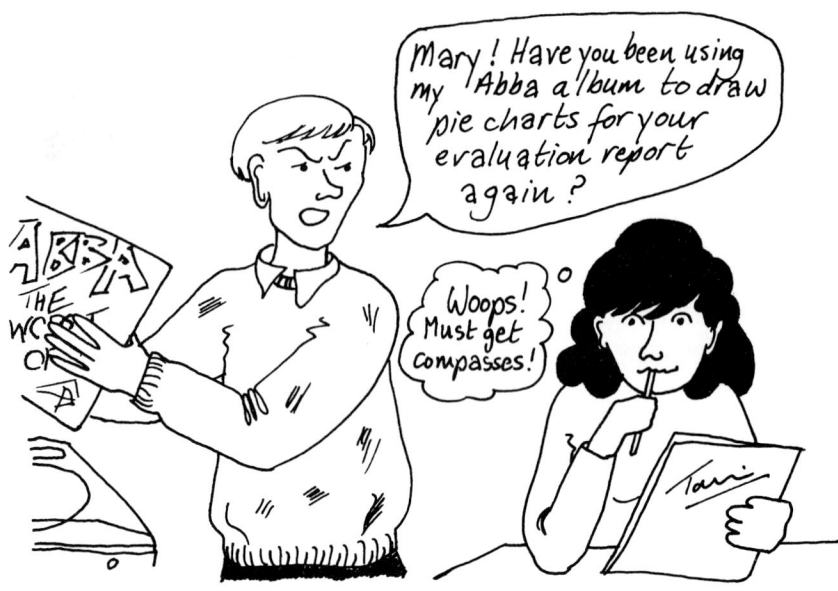

and qualitative data (see the appendix for more details relating to the analysis of questionnaires).

In most cases, it will be sufficient to analyse quantitative data descriptively.(8, 9, 14, 15) This may involve calculating averages, ranges, percentages and proportions. Descriptive statistics simply account for what is occurring in numerical terms. So, for example, when evaluating the use of a needle exchange system, an estimate may be made of the average number of people using the facility each week, or the percentage of users returning

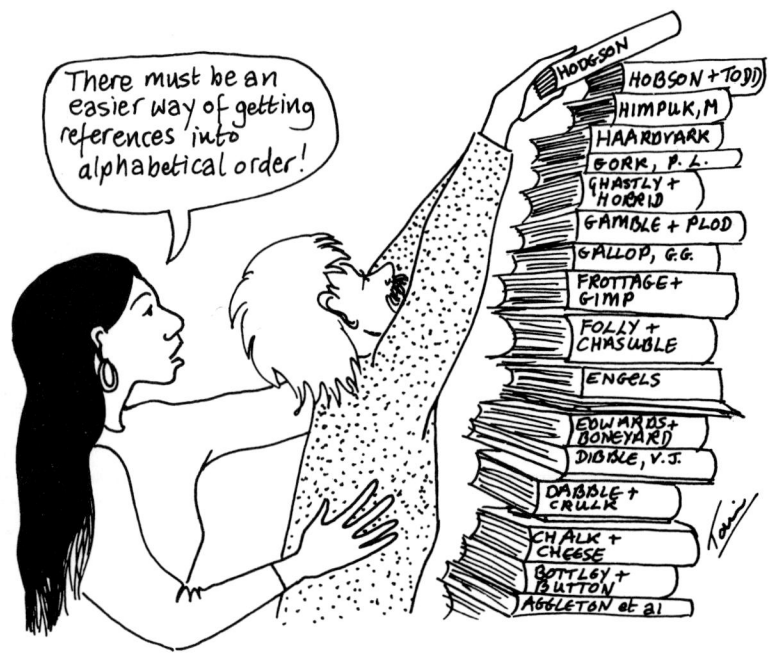

Producing evaluation reports 61

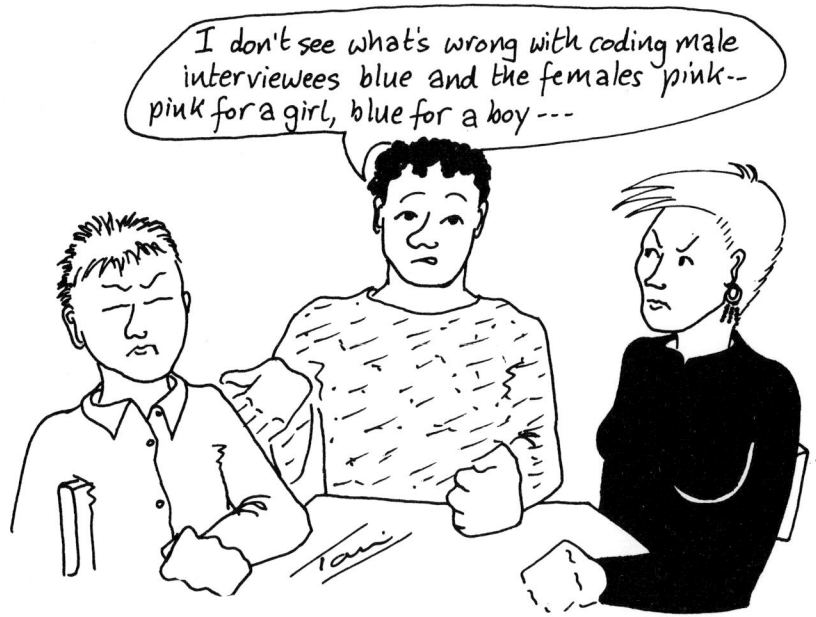

needles. The use of bar charts, pie charts, graphs and tables can be effective in conveying statistics in a clear and concise manner.

A large amount of qualitative information can be collected from interviews, case studies, records and observations, and it is important to organise this information into a workable order. It is useful to label the information carefully so that it is clear when it was collected, from whom and to what it relates. This may then be indexed for easy access.

Once the information has been organised, it may be

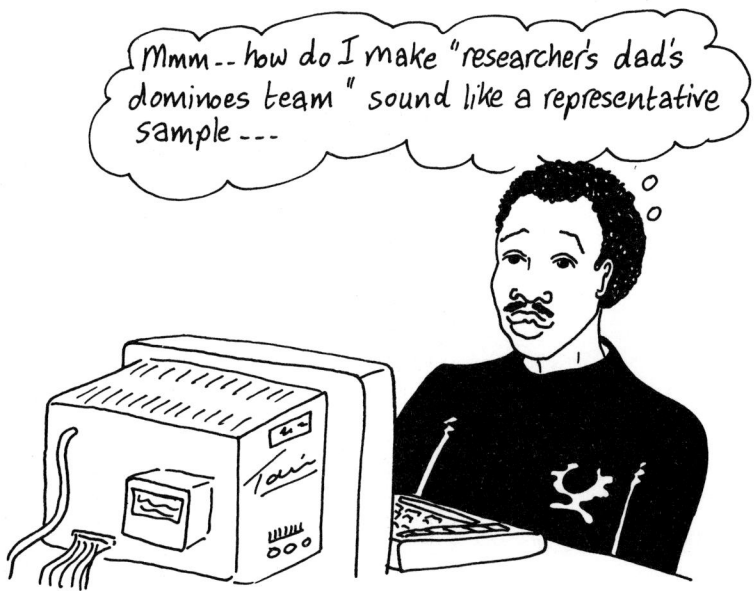

appropriate to develop a classification system. To do this, the information may be coded by number or colours according to categories or emerging themes. These might be, for example, what people learned from the activity, what they enjoyed, or what positive or negative criticisms were made. The uses to which these data are put will depend to a large extent on the objectives of the evaluation.

It is often best to present the analysis in as simple a form as possible, so that the results will be clear to all. It is also important to recognise any limits to the evaluation methods used. For example, if data have only been collected from a sample of those involved in an HIV/AIDS health promotion activity, it may be important to consider how the sample was selected and whether it is genuinely representative.

Interpreting results

Interpreting results involves identifying the implications and importance of a particular set of findings. This may be done by comparing the actual results with what was expected, or by identifying those aspects of the activity that seem to have particularly influenced its success or failure. Clearly, any inferences drawn should be logical and based on the facts.

To help to explain results, it may be important to involve other staff members, decision makers and participants. Any opposing ideas should be presented to give a balanced view, and it is important to realise that there is usually more than one way of interpreting a set of data. It may be necessary to state this explicitly in any evaluation report. The challenge lies in deciding which of the various interpretations better explains the evidence.

It is particularly important when interpreting information from a process evaluation to recognise that the views and activities of individuals, groups and even organisations are under scrutiny – the sensitivity of this kind of data is often underestimated. For example, it may be important to refer to past 'mistakes' so that these can be rectified and the activity developed accordingly in the future. It is essential that those involved in the activity have a chance to comment on any interpretation of the data that refers to their activities, views and responsibilities. These comments need to be given equal weight in relation to those of the evaluators, so that the evaluation is ultimately fair and honest.

Writing reports

It is good practice to prepare a written report of an evaluation, outlining the relevant findings. The first step when writing a report is to reconsider the questions and issues that were

Producing evaluation reports

formulated when planning the evaluation. It might be worth reconsidering, for example, exactly *why* the evaluation was undertaken, *who* the evaluation was for and *why* a particular type of evaluation was used. It is also important to consider *when* the findings will be needed and *who* the report is written for.

Exercise 18 **Report writing**

Aim To help you to consider the strengths and weaknesses of different kinds of report writing.

The following three reports on the same training workshop represent three styles of report writing, albeit with some exaggeration. What are the strengths and weaknesses of each style? (You may find it useful to refer back to the ST CRAVE mnemonic on pages 18–19.)

Report 1

Jo and Paul recently met up with a group of young people and spent an interesting evening talking about things that concerned them all. Everyone said that it had gone really well and they'd learnt lots about prejudices and AIDS. Some parts of the evening raised plenty of laughs, particularly the game with the courgettes. These proved to be in greater demand than the free condoms, even among the unexpected participants from the neighbouring rooms, and Mrs Cromarty, the organiser, was congratulated on her choice of refreshments.

Report 2

That the aetiology of cognitive behavioural modification among pubescent pre-entrants into the Registrar General's median classes (II–IV as defined by cumulative frequency rating of the occupational status of the head of household) may be dialectic rather than linear was corroborated by an experiment in non-didactic extra-curricular conferencing. By formative and summative means, Passons *et al.* have shown that the mean scores within the inter-quartile range of 11.4 young men, whose average pre-experimental familiarisation was 15.6666% at four hours and over, varied between 28.9 seconds and 0.196 hours. However, these figures do not take into account the anxiety-restorative function of intermittent symbolic-interactionist participative observation by the researchers' control group. Statistically significant, self-reporting revealed the criticality of positive-aural, tension-reduction techniques, particularly directly concomitant with accidental breakages. Unfortunately, these results cannot be generalised as the researchers failed to take into account control group interference factors.

Report 3

Greater Hemsham's Safer Sex Awareness Programme is now being piloted in youth clubs by youth and community outreach workers. The objectives are to increase knowledge of modes of HIV transmission, safer and unsafe sexual practices, to encourage young men to talk about sex, familiarisation with correct condom use, and identifying and challenging negative attitudes to HIV prevention. Jo Passons and Paul White co-facilitated a two-hour workshop at the Hemsham Vale Under 18s Club. This was attended by 14 boys aged 16–18 of whom 11 stayed to the end. While only two of the boys claimed to be sexually active, all but one had seen a condom, although only half of the group claimed to have ever opened a packet before. The workshop programme consisted of brief introductions, a pre-activity quiz to test knowledge of HIV infection routes, a warm-up exercise that involved listing different words for men's and women's genitals, a game to rate the safety of various sexual activities, an exercise to practise putting condoms on correctly (using courgettes to make it light-hearted) and a repeat of the quiz at the end. Discussion was encouraged throughout and the workers stayed for informal chats during the refreshment period at the end. On the basis of group discussion, informal feedback and facilitators' records, it would seem that the participants dealt with their initial embarrassment through laughter, and were able to identify and to address worries and confusions about the practice and relevance of safer sex to them. While attempts to disrupt the workshop by a neighbouring class detracted from the sense of trust and safety in the group, analysis of the quiz showed an average increase in understanding of transmission routes of 75%.

You are likely to find that while one report has been designed as a 'good example', there are strengths and weaknesses in each paragraph. Which strengths are a feature of your style of report writing? Do you tend towards any of the weaknesses you have identified?

There are several ways of writing an evaluation report. A 'formal' evaluation report will usually adopt the following format (16):

1. *Summary*: This is placed at the beginning of the report and

outlines briefly and concisely the main points to emerge from the evaluation.
2. *Introduction*: This may include an overview of the activity, detailing its aims and objectives. It may also place the activity within the wider organisational context and refer to similar projects. The rationale for the evaluation will also be outlined.
3. *Purpose/aim*: The purpose of the evaluation should be detailed here. This may include reference to some of the questions considered when planning the evaluation, such as who the evaluation is for, what is evaluated and when. This may involve justifying some of the decisions taken.
4. *Method*: The methods used in the evaluation should be described in detail, including the study design, the techniques used (questionnaires, interviews, monitoring records, etc.), how they were used, who was involved in the evaluation and how respondents were selected. It is also important to refer to the strengths and weaknesses of the methods employed, the problems faced and how these were overcome.
5. *Results*: This section details findings from any quantitative analysis and outlines the main themes emerging through qualitative analysis. It may include direct quotes of relevant comments made. This section may also include graphs, tables and bar charts, summarising trends in the data.
6. *Discussion and conclusion*: This section draws together the main findings of the evaluation to point to what has occurred in the activity and to explain why some aspects of the activity seemed to work better than others. It also discusses whether the activity achieved what it intended to.
7. *Recommendations*: These should be based on the evidence emerging from the evaluation and should suggest what is to be done in the future (i.e. the course of action), as well as indicate any changes or improvements that need to be made to the activity. There are several things to bear in mind here:

- Recommendations should be based on a logical interpretation of the findings.
- Recommendations should recognise that there may be several courses of action and each option should be presented to facilitate a considered choice.
- A clear distinction should be made between recommendations dealing with central issues and those dealing with secondary issues. Distinctions should also be made between recommendations that can be

achieved in the short term and those that are more likely to be attained in the long term.
- Recommendations should, where possible, be written in conjunction with senior staff or planning teams who may be involved in the implementation of the recommendations, and also stakeholders and others who have an interest in the activity.

It is important to ensure that the recommendations are well balanced and reflect not only the findings of the evaluation, but also take into account the aims and nature of the HIV/AIDS health promotion activity.

8. *References*: This section should list any publications, articles and reports that have been quoted or cited in the evaluation report.
9. *Appendices*: This may include any materials used (e.g. a copy of a questionnaire or interview schedule). It may also include a list of people interviewed.

It may be that the evaluation method used and the type of information collected does not lend itself to a structured report. If there are several components to an activity, and consequently to the evaluation, it may be feasible to split the report into sections, each focusing on a particular theme. For example, in an evaluation of a series of HIV/AIDS training courses carried out over a twelve-month period, the evaluation report may be structured to include (a) a general introduction; (b) a section on the structure and organisation of the training courses (how long each course ran, what it involved, what its aims were and how it was facilitated); (c) a section on the training courses in the context of the organisation in which they were run, how they were funded and their rationale; (d) a section on the participants (who took part, what their backgrounds were, how many took part and how many were invited on the course); (e) a section on how participants felt about the activity, and also about how others involved in the activity felt (e.g. facilitators and administrators); and (f) a section on the outcomes of the activity both in the long term and the short term. The report may end with conclusions and recommendations. Alternatively, only a short report may be required, discussing some of these issues but in the form of a chronological 'story' or diary that includes a record of achievements, problems, comments and thoughts expressed. In each case, the style of the report will depend on who the report is for and the type of information that is collected.

Exercise 19 **Putting an evaluation report together**

Aim To provide practice in writing evaluation reports.

Choose one HIV/AIDS health promotion activity from the following list:

- Outreach work within Vietnamese communities.
- A women's sexual assertion training course.
- A leaflet promoting safer injecting practices.
- A support group to promote healthy loving for lesbian and gay teenagers.
- An activity from your own experience.

Imagine that this work is being evaluated and that you are responsible for briefing the person who will write the report. Answer the following questions, making up and supplying details as you consider appropriate:

- Who is the report for?
- What types of quantitative information have been collected?
- What types of qualitative information have been collected?
- How formal/informal does the report need to be?
- What sections do you want included in the report? Plan it, either linearly or using patterned notes (see pages 2–3).

Conclusions

Analysing and interpreting information and writing an evaluation report constitute the penultimate stage in the evaluation process. It is important that report writing is done sensitively, as the evaluation report can often be the 'public face' not only of the evaluation itself, but also of the HIV/AIDS health promotion activity as a whole. When analysing data and writing reports, it is vitally important to bear in mind who the evaluation is for and how the findings will be used.

The final stage of the evaluation process involves using the evaluation findings. These may be used to influence and to improve future work practice, and also as a means of sharing experiences.

In addition, they may be used to attract future funding. Chapter 6 considers some of the ways in which information from an evaluation can be used.

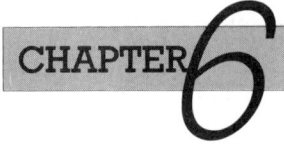
CHAPTER 6

Using evaluation

- Influencing policy
- Influencing personal and professional life

Introduction

HIV infection and AIDS have presented many opportunities for health promotion. Knowing the facts about HIV transmission and practising safer behaviour are presently recognised as the only means of guarding against infection. HIV/AIDS workers are only too aware of this and are attempting to increase knowledge and to promote behaviour change in a variety of ways. In striving to do this, they face a formidable set of challenges. First, knowledge of HIV/AIDS is constantly growing. Second, HIV/AIDS workers have to be ever sensitive to the social, emotional and political aspects of their work. Third, their actions are limited by the existing knowledge about how best to encourage behaviour change. In this context, evaluating HIV/AIDS health promotion activities is not merely an academic issue, but is also of fundamental importance in planning and developing better and more appropriate services. It is also important in ensuring that the information gathered, and the understanding gained, are shared and disseminated.

Evaluation is also concerned with values such as accountability, open discussion and decision making, and the rational distribution of resources. However, while evaluation has enormous potential as a tool for empowerment, it is not a magical answer to the problems of scarcity of resources, oppressive power relations, people's occasional capacity to misrepresent and to justify the worst practices, and the hidden ways in which pressures can be channelled and exerted through institutions. Evaluation does not neutralise the risk that feelings of insecurity, fear, anxiety and competitiveness may discourage some people in some organisations from pursuing full accountability at all times.

Nonetheless, the potential benefits of using evaluation as a tool far outweigh the risks. Evaluation enables services to be improved and campaigns to be made more effective. It improves communication and challenges all stakeholders to greater accountability and power sharing. Ultimately, then, evaluation is an essential instrument for those committed to good policy and practice, effective service delivery and honouring the best interests of service users. As such, it is vitally important that it is used sensitively, effectively and with confidence.

It is important that lessons are learned from past experience, and that knowledge gained from different HIV/AIDS health promotion activities is used in the development of future work. It is important, too, that responses to HIV/AIDS are based on a thorough understanding of the strengths and limitations of existing health promotion approaches. This can only occur once the challenge of evaluation has been met, and only if the results of an evaluation are well used.

Influencing policy

Although the evaluation of HIV/AIDS health promotion activities presents a challenge, it is, more importantly, necessary to ensure that HIV/AIDS work becomes increasingly effective, and that monetary and political support for it continues. Ultimately, a key requirement of evaluation is to provide policy makers with information that relates to the use of resources that have been invested. By using the information from an evaluation future decisions about the allocation of scarce resources can be made on a more rational and well-informed basis.

It is reasonable to expect that if an evaluation shows an activity to have been successful, then that activity might be repeated elsewhere. The aim here is for the evaluation to describe not only a particular activity, but also the specific circumstances under which it was implemented. The information collected during an evaluation can thereby be applied usefully in the planning of new and future activities.

It is essential, however, that what can be learnt from an evaluation is not undermined by factors such as inadequate reporting mechanisms or by the level of work pressure, which is so often faced by workers. Such a situation perpetuates a culture of crisis management in which too little time is allocated to strategic thinking. Good evaluation should form the basis on which to develop future planning, and should be able to address and to reformulate policy questions relating to HIV/AIDS.

At the outset of an evaluation therefore, it is important to consider and to develop mechanisms by which the findings of the evaluation can be discussed, not only with those involved in the activity, but also with stakeholders and funders. It is also important that the level of institutional support for the activity and for the evaluation itself is scrutinised before and during the evaluation. It may be necessary to include those 'higher' in the institutional hierarchy in the evaluation, so that the findings and recommendations are not, and cannot, be ignored. After rising to

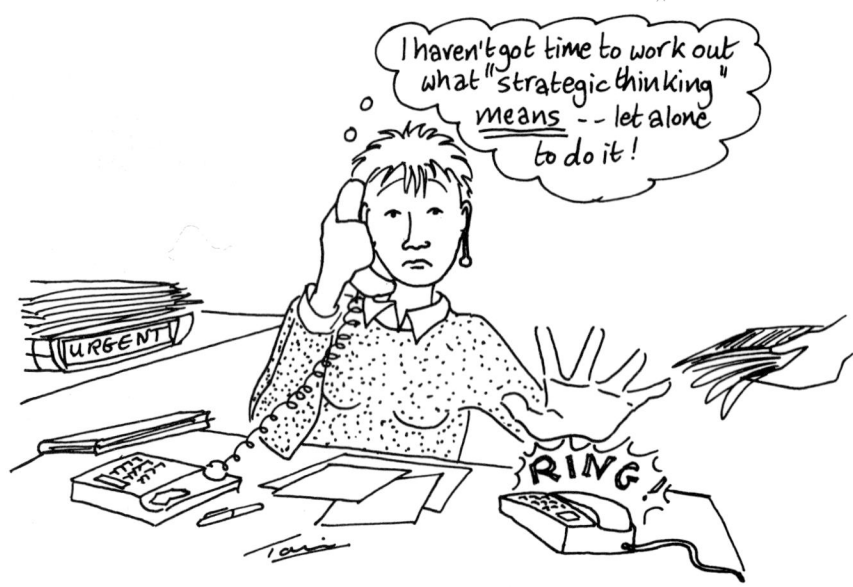

the challenge of carrying out an evaluation, it would be a shame to fall at the last hurdle.

Influencing personal and professional life

Evaluation can be used not only to facilitate planning and to influence policy development, but also to enhance self and group development. An evaluation sets out to analyse a situation, it investigates the context and constraints surrounding an activity, and it provides an understanding of how the activity works. By gaining an insight into the context and process of their project, workers are likely to become involved in a process of self-empowerment.

The importance of evaluation to those involved in HIV/AIDS work should not be underestimated, since it is a process that allows workers to understand and to redefine their work roles, enables their work and the work of others to be valued and validated, and gives workers the opportunity to reflect on what they are doing. Negative or critical findings should therefore be treated in a way that allows potential problems to be confronted positively, to develop the activity, rather than in a way that encourages recrimination or blame.

It may be useful to develop a mechanism by which information from an evaluation can be 'fed back' to those involved in an HIV/AIDS health promotion activity. This could take the form of a workshop that allows time for the findings to be discussed and for grievances, if any, to be aired. Ultimately, such an occasion might act as a team-building exercise. It will also be important as an impetus for future action planning.

Using evaluation 71

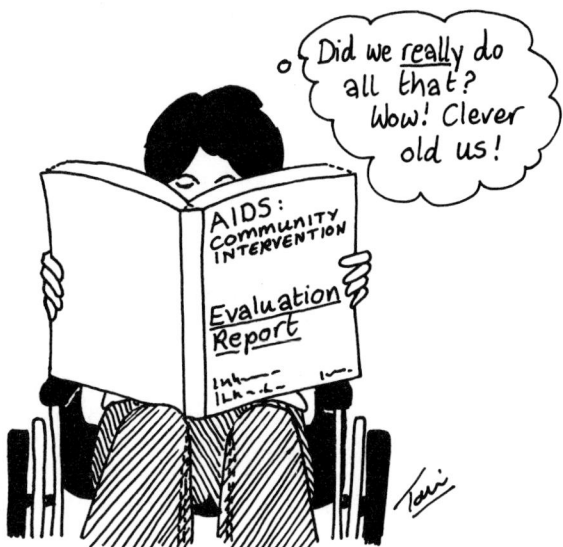

Conclusions

It is essential that the findings of an evaluation are put to good use. The whole process of evaluation is invalidated if it is not intimately linked to the development and planning of HIV/AIDS activities and services. It is important therefore that careful consideration is given to how evaluation findings can be fed back to those involved in the activity, and to how any recommendations can be implemented.

Finally, it is important to 'evaluate the evaluation'. Here, time should be given to considering how successful the evaluation was, by asking questions such as 'Did it achieve what it set out to achieve?', 'How was the evaluation received?', 'Did it miss vital information?' and 'What lessons can be learnt for the next time?'

Exercise 20 **Final self-assessment**

Aim To help you to assess what you have learned from this resource.

Complete this exercise when you have finished studying this book and you feel you have extracted all the information you need.

- Which sections, if any, have you studied?
- Since first using this resource, what factors have influenced your approach to evaluation?

Without looking back at your initial self-assessment (see pages 4–6), rate yourself on the following criteria. Date and keep a copy of your response.

A. Grade your current impressions of yourself as an evaluator on a scale from 0 (very poor) through 5 (adequate) to 10 (excellent) in the following areas.

  (i)   Overall knowledge of evaluation. ☐

  (ii) Knowing how to carry out evaluation and knowing which approaches to use in specific situations. ☐

  (iii) Confidence that you have the necessary understanding to meet the evaluation needs of your present post. ☐

B. How would you rate your attitude to evaluation on a scale of 0 (very low) through 5 (sometimes useful) to 10 (essential)? ☐

Has your attitude to evaluation changed in any way, and if so, how?

C. Taking no more than ten minutes, make patterned notes around the central topic of evaluation (see pages 2–3).

Before completing the final part of this exercise, take a break so that you can return to it with some detachment.

D. Compare your initial self-assessment on pages 4–6 with your final self-assessment here.

- What differences, if any, do you notice in your various ratings and the content/form of your patterned notes?
- What do you think may account for these differences?

Appendix

- **Constructing a questionnaire**
- **Wording questions**
- **Analysing the results**

Constructing a questionnaire

When constructing a questionnaire, there are several points to bear in mind.(17) First, the questions must be designed so that they are easy to understand. The vocabulary used needs to be familiar to respondents and the questions need to be clearly worded. Ambiguous and unfamiliar words will make questions hard to answer. Second, in most cases the questionnaires should be anonymous and confidential. It is unlikely that respondents will answer sensitive questions honestly if there is a possibility of the information being traced. Third, the structure and length of the questionnaire should be designed to keep the respondent's interest. The first few questions should be interesting and easy to answer, while the questionnaire as a whole should not be too long.

With these principles in mind, it is important to consider the types of questions to use. The questionnaire may include *open-ended questions* or *pre-coded* questions. Open-ended questions may be asked when a detailed answer is required or when it is not possible to foresee all the potential range of answers. For example, 'What do you understand by the term 'safer sex'?' Although open-ended questions require more time to analyse, they may produce a depth of information that is not possible with pre-coded questions. However, respondents may find open-ended questions difficult to answer, and so it is often wise to include a selection of both open-ended and pre-coded questions.

Pre-coded questions can be used in several ways. They may take the simple format of either 'yes/no' or 'true/false' questions, which may be useful when assessing people's knowledge of and attitude towards HIV/AIDS. For example:

HIV can be transmitted by (mark YES or NO):
    Vaginal sex   YES ☐ NO ☐
    Using public toilets   YES ☐ NO ☐
    Kissing   YES ☐ NO ☐
    Sharing cups and glasses YES ☐ NO ☐

State whether each of the following statements is TRUE or FALSE:

There is no known cure for AIDS.	TRUE ☐	FALSE ☐
Using a condom is 100% safe.	TRUE ☐	FALSE ☐
AIDS is mainly a problem for gay men.	TRUE ☐	FALSE ☐
HIV can be transmitted from mother to baby during pregnancy.	TRUE ☐	FALSE ☐

A four- or five-point scale may be used to give a more comprehensive assessment of attitudes. For example:

People with AIDS should notify their work colleagues of the fact:

Strongly agree ☐
Agree ☐
Neither agree nor disagree ☐
Disagree ☐
Strongly disagree ☐

This may be presented diagrammatically:

Agree | | | | | Disagree

0   /

Alternatively, a semantic differential scale asks people to choose a point on a scale of opposites to indicate their feelings:

Good |___|___|___|___ Bad

Finally, it may be useful to present the questionnaire as a 'quiz'. Although the same type of question might be asked, respondents might find a quiz more fun than a questionnaire, and may therefore be more willing to take part.

Wording questions

When constructing a questionnaire, it is important to ensure that questions are not worded in a way that encourages biased or misleading answers. For example, a poorly written question can assume that a respondent already holds a particular point of view. So, it is best to preface a question such as 'What is it that you like about this safer sex leaflet?' with another that first asks 'Do you like or dislike this safer sex leaflet?' Other more subtle kinds of leading question may suggest to respondents that there is only one socially acceptable answer to a given question. It is important when working with HIV/AIDS that all views are considered, even if they are felt to be offensive.

Questions that use negatives are sometimes difficult to understand, especially if the respondent is being asked to agree or disagree with a given statement. For example, 'People with AIDS should not avoid kissing' may be a confusing statement for some respondents to answer. It is also important to avoid ambiguous or misleading terms. Terms such as 'having sex', 'taking drugs' and 'sleeping with a man' do not have a uniform meaning to all respondents. Finally, it is important to avoid double-barrelled questions, such as 'Can HIV be transmitted via vaginal and anal intercourse?' Respondents may have different feelings towards vaginal and anal intercourse that cannot be reflected in a single answer.

Analysing the results

Pre-coded questions can be analysed in several ways. Simple 'yes/no' questions may be analysed by counting the number of people who have replied yes or no to each statement and expressing this as a percentage. If pre- and post-tests are used, the percentage of correct answers in the pre-test can be compared to the percentage of correct post-test answers. For example, for the question 'HIV can be transmitted by ...', the following results may occur:

HIV can be transmitted by:	% Correct		
	Pre-test	Post-test	Difference
Vaginal sex	73.3	78.0	4.7
Using public toilets	40.5	70.9	30.4
Kissing	61.3	87.1	25.8
Sharing cups and glasses	25.7	65.0	39.3

Answers to a question using a five-point scale can be summarised in a similar way by using a tally method – this is the *frequency distribution*. For example, from a sample of 20 people, answers to the question 'People with AIDS should notify their work colleagues of the fact' may be summarised as follows:

Strongly agree	Agree	Neither	Disagree	Strongly disagree
||	++++	|||	++++	 ||	++++

This may then be expressed as a percentage; for example, 35% of respondents disagreed with the statement, or 55% of respondents disagreed or strongly disagreed with the statement, while only 35% strongly agreed or agreed with the statement. When several questions on a questionnaire are summarised in this way, a particular pattern of response may be revealed.

This is the most elementary means of statistical description, although often the analysis of survey data does not go much beyond the use of descriptive statistics. More complex analytical methods of analysis require careful planning and consideration to be given to issues such as sampling methods and the use of tests of significance and correlation.(15, 18)

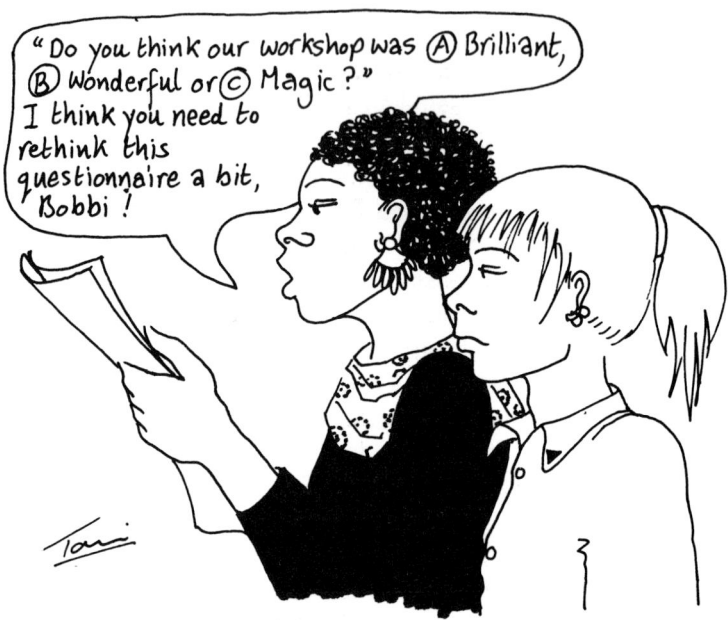

References

1. World Health Organisation (1989). *Monitoring of National AIDS Prevention and Control Programmes – Guiding Principles*, WHO AIDS Series 4. WHO, Geneva.
2. Kapila, Mukesh (1990). *Introductory Concepts in the Evaluation of AIDS Health Promotion Programmes*, AIDS Programme Paper 7. Health Education Authority, London.
3. Scott, Sue (1992). 'Evaluation may change your life but it won't solve all your problems', in *Does it Work? Perspectives on the Evaluation of HIV/AIDS Health Promotion*, ed. Peter Aggleton, Andrea Young, Diane Moody, Mukesh Kapila and Maryan Pye. Health Education Authority, London.
4. Feuerstein, M. (1986). *Partners in Evaluation*, Macmillan, London.
5. Prout, Allan (1992). 'Illumination, collaboration, facilitation, negotiation: evaluating the MESMAC Project', in *Does it Work? Perspectives on the Evaluation of HIV/AIDS Health Promotion*, ed. Peter Aggleton, Andrea Young, Diane Moody, Mukesh Kapila and Maryan Pye. Health Education Authority, London.
6. Basch, C. E. (1987). 'Focus group interview: an underutilized research technique for improving theory and practice in health education', *Health Education Quarterly*, winter, pp. 410–48.
7. Aggleton, Peter (1989). 'Evaluating health education about AIDS', in *AIDS: Social Representations, Social Practices*, ed. Peter Aggleton, Graham Hart and Peter Davies. Falmer Press, Lewes.
8. de Vaus, D. A. (1990). *Surveys in Social Research*, chapter 4. Unwin Hyman, London.
9. Bryman, Alan and Cramer, Duncan (1990). *Quantitative Data Analysis for Social Scientists*, chapter 6. Routledge, London.
10. Dixon, Beverly, Bouma, Gary and Atkinson, G. B. J. (1987). *A Handbook of Social Science Research*, chapter 7. Oxford University Press, Oxford.
11. de Vaus, D. A. (1990). *Surveys in Social Research*, chapters 6 and 7. Unwin Hyman, London.
12. Hitchcock, Graham and Hughes, David. (1990). *Research and the Teacher: Qualitative Introduction to School Based Research*, chapter 4. Routledge, London.
13. Godfrey, Christine and Tolley, Keith (1992). 'An economic

approach to the evaluation of HIV/AIDS health education programmes', in *Does it Work? Perspectives on the Evaluation of HIV/AIDS Health Promotion*, ed. Peter Aggleton, Andrea Young, Diane Moody, Mukesh Kapila and Maryan Pye. Health Education Authority, London.

14. Dixon, Beverly, Bouma, Gary and Atkinson, G. B. J. (1987). *A Handbook of Social Science Research*, chapters 9 and 10. Oxford University Press, Oxford.
15. Youngman, M. B. (1979). *Analysing Social and Educational Research Data*. McGraw-Hill, Maidenhead.
16. Clarkson, J. and Nutbeam, D. (1989). *Evaluation Handbook*, Heartbeat Wales Technical Report 19. Health Promotion Authority for Wales, Cardiff.
17. Hoinville, G. *et al.* (1985). *Survey Research Practice*. Gower, Aldershot.
18. Moser, C. A. and Kalton, G. (1981). *Survey Methods in Social Investigation*. Heinemann, London.

Further reading

Whitehead, M. and Tones, K. (1991). *Avoiding the Pitfalls: Notes on the Planning and Implementation of Health Education Strategies and the Special Role of the HEA*. Health Education Authority, London.
Tones, K., Tilford, S. and Robinson, Y. (1991). *Health Education – Effectiveness and Efficiency*. Chapman & Hall, London.